SOUTHPORT

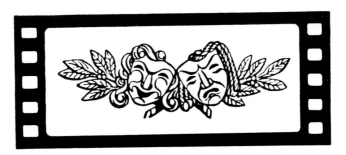

Stage&Screen

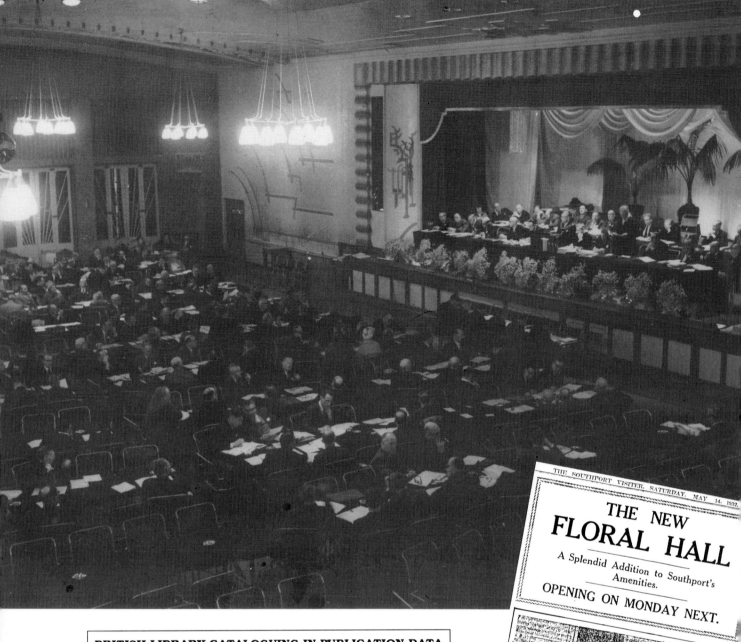

THE SOUTHPORT VISITER, SATURDAY, MAY 14, 1932.

THE NEW
FLORAL HALL

A Splendid Addition to Southport's
Amenities.

OPENING ON MONDAY NEXT.

BRITISH LIBRARY CATALOGUING IN PUBLICATION DATA
Ackroyd, Harold
    Southport stage & screen
    1. Merseyside (England). Recreation buildings. History
    1. Title
    791.43094275

    ISBN 0-9514235-0-9

First printed 1991

SOUTHPORT STAGE & SCREEN
By Harold Ackroyd

Produced, printed and published by
Amber Valley Print Centre

ISBN 0 9514235 0 9

The art deco interior of the Floral
Hall.
Photo: Metropolitan Borough of
Sefton (D. Taylor, Attractions
Department)

SOUTHPORT

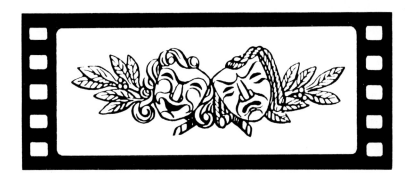

Stage&Screen

Harold Ackroyd

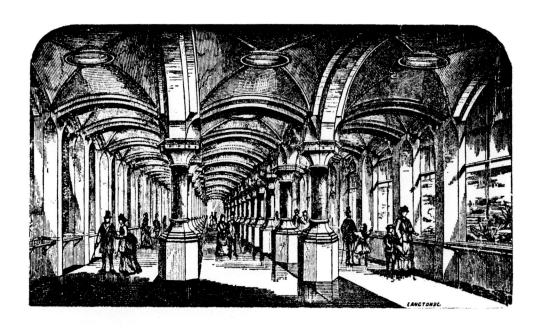

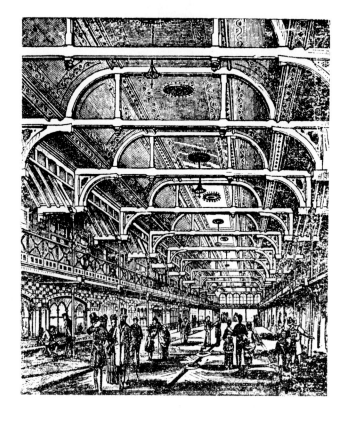

The Winter Gardens complex.
Top: The Aquarium, like the crypt
of a cathedral, was in the basement
beneath the Promenade Hall.
Above: The Promenade Hall which
joined the Conservatory and the
Pavilion.
Right: The Conservatory.
See page 9 for the location of the
various sections of the Winter
Gardens.
Drawings: Geoff Wright

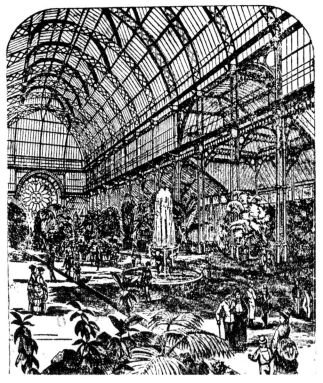

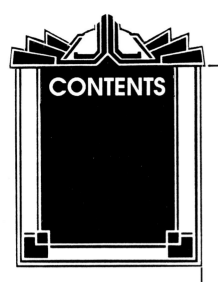

CONTENTS

ACKNOWLEDGEMENTS

The excellent coverage of Southport entertainments in the town's newspaper the *Southport Visitor*, has provided an invaluable source of information during the research for this book, but for other less easily obtainable information, sincere thanks to Mr. Ashby Ball, Chartered Surveyor, and Mr. Leslie Houghton of Southport, without whose assistance much would have remained undiscovered. Thanks also to the staff of the Southport reference library, Mrs Janet Jenkins, Sefton local historian, Mr. Roger Hull, Crosby reference library, and Mr. Harry Hosker, Building Design Partnership, Preston.

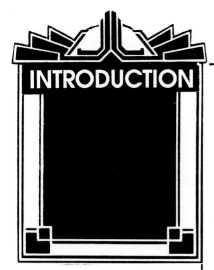

INTRODUCTION

Although the theatre in Southport enjoyed a long and memorable heyday in the Victorian era (1837 to 1901) it is recorded that the town's first theatrical venture was in the years between 1821 and 1825, a temporary theatre in a building at the rear of the present Scarisbrick Hotel on Lord Street. This hazardously-constructed wooden theatre opened at the end of October 1821 with a presentation on two successive nights of *The Honeymoon*, a comedy in five acts by the dramatist John Tobin, attended by a crowded and fashionable audience. This temporary theatre was soon replaced by a more permanent one in Upper King Street on the upper storey of the Assembly Rooms.

In 1845 Butterworth's Theatre was opened behind the Union Hotel, to be followed a year later by the Royal Albion Theatre, and the Town Hall was regularly used for theatrical purposes after its opening on 1st June 1853. Butterworth's Theatre, stated to have a distinguished patronage, was badly damaged by a heavy gale during the summer of 1845, but after repairs was able to persevere with its schedules of rather heavy Victorian melodramas. The Royal Albion Theatre, opened in a pavilion in front of the Union Hotel, was described as a place of historic amusement and attracted large audiences.

The Royal Museum in Portland Street was the enterprise of William Newby, opened on 19th May 1863, and by the autumn of 1868 it had become the Royal Music Hall which could be hired for concerts etc. Gladstone spoke there in 1868, the year he became Prime Minister. In March 1872 a theatrical licence was granted and it became known as Southport's Bijou Theatre, but unsupported by public money as the other theatrical enterprises, its career was hazardous. Under the control of Julian Malvern in 1874 it was re-named the Vaudeville Theatre, but did not prosper due to increasing competition from the Pavilion in the new Winter Gardens complex opened on 16th September of that year, and a few years later there was a further change of use to a skating rink.

1874 was indeed among the most important years in the entertainment history of Southport, for not only did it see the opening of the Cambridge Hall for concerts and theatrical purposes, but also the vast and wonderful leisure complex named the Winter Gardens. It was there in the Pavilion, originally a concert hall, that theatrical events first commenced as a permanent attraction during the first half of 1878. The great variety of entertainment ranged from the operas of Carl Rosa and D'Oyly Carte to dramatic plays with the great actor, Henry Irving. During the next fifteen years the Winter Gardens' shows became so popular that special trains were run to the adjacent Lancashire & Yorkshire Railway's Lord Street station.

But great as had been the success of the theatre in Victorian Southport, this did not reach its peak until 1891 when the Opera House was opened by the Winter Gardens company, and was for many years Southport's most popular place of entertainment, staging the best in drama, musical comedy and farce with the most famous actors and actresses.

During the last years of the century, as in many towns and cities throughout the country, the new novelty attraction - animated pictures were shown. The first exhibition was at the Winter Gardens, Coronation Hall on 7th July 1896 with half-hourly performances from 3pm to 5pm and 7pm to 9pm. Advertised as "The Talk of the Town" and "The Wonder of the Age" it was reported that the life-size pictures were shown by Messrs J.F. Tester, AIEE and W.A. Robbins operating a projector known as the Kineopticon, in a marvellously clear and natural manner. For an admission charge of 6d, the films, "as exhibited before H.R.H. the Prince of Wales" were entitled, *Arrival of a Margate Steamer, The Sea at Dover, Prize Fight, The Boxing Kangaroo, The Derby, Children on the Sands at Yarmouth* and *Feeding a Tiger*.

The former Leyland Arcade behind Boothroyd's store on Lord Street, opened in 1898, was another early location for film shows, first listed in the town's directory of 1900 as The Bioscope, 42 Leyland Arcade by the Mutoscope and Biograph Syndicate Ltd. These were continued until 1909 under the control of several other companies. Leased to the MacNagthen Vaudeville circuit in 1908, the Pier Pavilion presented variety supported by Raymond's Bio-Tableaux (Matt Raymond's silent pictures) as the Whitsuntide attractions, and in the same year, Frenchman Leon Gaumont's device, the Chronophone, linking a projector with a phonograph was used for pictures with sound at the Temperance Hall.

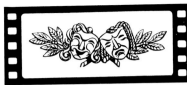

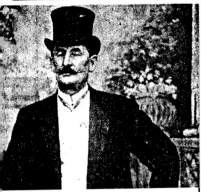

Alf Wilden, one of the first to show "moving pictures" on Merseyside.
Photo: *Southport Visitor*

There are apparently two claimants to the opening of Southport's first cinema - Alf Wilden and George Berthold Samuelson, but whilst the former's fairground show in 1908 was a year before his rival's Electric Theatre, this it would appear more justified the description of a cinema. In the summer of 1908 Alf Wilden, a blacksmith turned travelling Showman, opened a boxing booth in the fairground, but this was soon succeeded by the Bioscope Theatre, for which the iron-framed, wooden structure was built in sections by Alf in his back-yard at Banastre Road. Erected on the fairground, the building had a stage in front bearing the name in large painted letters "Wilden's Up-To-Date Cinematograph" upon which a "dancing girl named Annie, a chocolate coloured coon and a clown" performed with music by an organ to attract the crowds. Then Alf in evening dress and top hat would tell those assembled about the film show, persuading them to step inside for a few pence, to see the half-hour long programmes featuring a Wild West film and a drama or a comedy. These were shown with a hand-cranked projector by one of Alf's sons, Jack Wilden, formerly one of the boxers.

"Bertie" Samuelson, as he was known, opened the Victoria Hall, London Street, as the Electric Theatre on 25th November 1909 advertising "The Latest and Most Up-To-Date Pictures" at 8pm daily with admission at 3d, 6d and 1/- and children attending the first Saturday matinee on 27th November were to pay reduced prices of 2d, 3d and 6d and be presented with a toy! `Mr. Samuelson also opened a film hire business at King's Chambers, Tulketh Street in 1910, then following a move to Birmingham opened the Worton Hall film studios at Isleworth, Middlesex, in 1914, later becoming a pioneer film producer of the silent era.

Only six months after the opening of the Electric Theatre, Southport's first purpose built cinema, the Picturedrome was opened on Lord Street, closely followed by the Picture Palace in 1911. In 1913 were added the Empire and the Picture House, and by the time the Palladium opened in January 1914, Southport was regarded in the film industry as a first class town, especially since all the cinemas were granted licences for Sunday opening. It was quite fitting therefore that Southport should be among the first locations in the country for the screening of Edison's Kinetophone Talking Pictures, which were presented at the Picture House, Nevill Street for a season commencing Christmas 1913.

In addition to the attractions of concerts and ice skating, dancing increased in popularity as a leisure activity with the opening of the Winter Gardens ballroom in 1902, but it was during the years 1925 to 1929 that Southport became known as the dancing mecca of the North-West with the magnificent ballroom named the Palais de Danse, where Billy Cotton's was the first resident band. Thereafter from 1932, the Floral Hall included a dance floor among its attractions.

Despite the closure and demolition of the entire Winter Gardens complex, the town's varied selection of entertainment was continued in the thirties. The new sound films, or "talkies" as they were known, had been given an early showing at the Scala Cinema, which opened with *The Singing Fool* featuring Al Jolson, in April 1929. The new Palladium opened with cine-variety in 1930 and the following year the choice of 'Live' entertainment increased with the re-opening of the Pier Pavilion Theatre. In 1932 the Floral Hall included a dance floor among its attractions, and the year also saw the replacing of the Opera House by the Garrick Theatre. The Southport Dramatic Club opened the Little Theatre in 1937, and by the end of 1938 the addition of two super-cinemas had increased the number in the town to eight.

Although by the eighties the number of entertainment situations decreased considerably, this was almost entirely accounted for by cinema closures, which left the Cannon 1 & 2 the only surviving commercial cinemas, although films are still occasionally presented at the council-owned Southport Theatre and the Arts Centre, whilst the Little Theatre continues entirely as a 'live' theatre with plays performed by the Southport Dramatic Club, and the Floral Hall offers a variety of 'live' entertainment, concerts and dancing.

At this time, near to the end of the decade, Southport continues to present, for a town of its size, an above average range of entertainment.

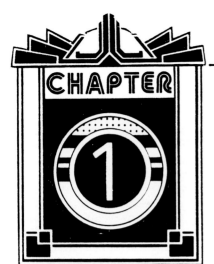

CHAPTER 1

WINTER GARDENS, Lord Street, Southport

In 1874 eight acres of Southport became an all year round resort with the opening on 16th September of the wonderful entertainment complex known as the Winter Gardens. The enterprise of Walter Smith, four times Mayor of Southport, this has been described as the most beautiful collection of buildings that ever graced the Southport skyline and the most interesting place the town has ever known, offering everything that then could be envisaged by way of entertainment.

The Lord Street frontage was originally occupied by two conservatories and an elaborate stone carriage port with arched entrance-ways from which a 15ft. wide grand staircase led up through landscaped gardens to the enclosed Promenade Hall with external verandahs and terraces. Extending across the present Kingsway, this was 170ft. long and 44ft. in width and resembled an ancient banqueting hall with colonnades supporting galleries below the hammer-beam ceiling at a height of 80ft., whilst other features were quaint windows set within a line of archways and longitudinal seats along the side walls. This entrance hall linked the 180ft. by 80ft. "Crystal Palace" style conservatory, stated to be the largest in England, with the Pavilion, a 2,500 concert hall with high arched ceiling supported by patterned steel girders, below which pairs of columns extended up from the surrounding first-floor gallery. There was an elegant proscenium and on the stage, the first entertainments were concerts twice daily by the thirty-piece Winter Gardens Orchestra.

At the opposite end of the entrance hall the conservatories contained a great variety of tropical trees, plants and flowers, a waterfall and an aviary of exotic birds amidst great glass walls festooned with creepers and curtained with foliage. The full extent of the Winter Gardens at ground level was repeated in the basement with two immense refreshment rooms under the Pavilion, whilst below the Promenade and Conservatory was an extensive Aquarium in which the vaulted ceiling was supported by massive white stone columns. 23 fish tanks were set in the walls and others supported on pillars so that they could be viewed on all sides. There was also a tank 66ft. long for large fish, also seal and crocodile pools.

The Winter Gardens from the Promenade. The Pavilion, later the Empire and then the Scala, is on the left and the "Crystal Palace" style Conservatory on the right. Between the two is the Promenade Hall. The building to the left of the photo is the Royal Hotel. The buildings on the ten acre Winter Gardens site included the Opera House, the Conservatory, the Aquarium, the Promenade Hall, the Pavilion, the Coronation Hall and the Circus.
Photo: Geoff Wright

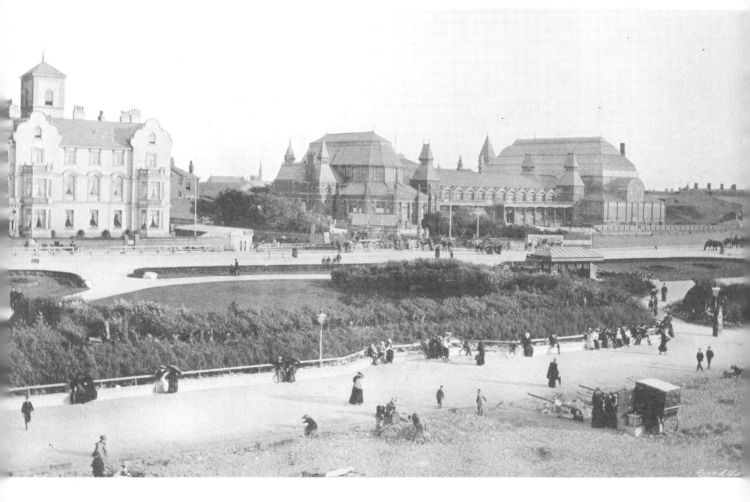

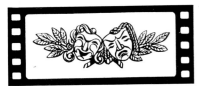

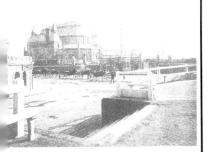

A simplified plan (not to scale) showing the various parts of the Winter Gardens. The dotted lines show the position of the present Kingsway. The Opera House site and entrance to the Pavilion is now the Top Rank bingo club (see chapter 17) and the Pavilion/Empire/Scala site is now the Safeway supermarket car park. The remainder of the site is being developed (1990) as the Winter Gardens Shopping Centre.
Plan: Amber Valley Print Centre

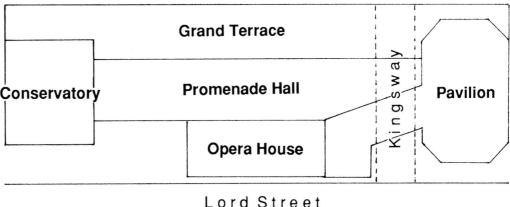

Beach

Promenade

Grand Terrace

Conservatory   Promenade Hall   Kingsway   Pavilion

Opera House

Lord Street

Along the sea frontage of the Winter Gardens was the Grand Terrace, 500ft. in length, below which the croquet lawn and sunken gardens were surrounded by a high wall to shelter the plants from the sea winds.

During the 1880s the conservatories on Lord Street were replaced by a roller rink, and an iron and wooden circus building was erected in the gardens between the rink and the Pavilion. Restricted stage space at the Pavilion resulted in the building of the Opera House in 1891 on the Lord Street site of the skating rink. The new theatre was considered one of architect Frank Matcham's masterpieces, and at a cost of £20,000, a large sum at that time, it had a seating capacity of 1,,492 with boxes, stalls, dress circle,upper circle and gallery. The flamboyant facade featured arched windows, curved gables with scrollwork pinnacles and Islamic cupolas, whilst below the full width iron and glass verandah supported along the front by ornamental iron pillars, shops flanked the main entrance. The auditorium had excellent sight lines and acoustics, and a 50ft. deep stage on which were presented operas, musicals and plays by companies from London's West End. The opening attraction on 7 September 1891 was the Haymarket success, *The Dancing Girl* by M. Van Biene's company including Miss Katie Vaughan, to which admission prices ranged from 6d to 5/- with boxes at 15/- and a guinea.

Following the winding-up of the Winter Gardens company in 1901 the complex came under the control of North Marine Entertainments, proprietor and general manager Gilbert Rogers. Roller and ice skating rinks were added and the sunken gardens along the sea frontage replaced by a boating lake and switchback railway. A Christmas attraction for 1902, Edison's World Famous Animated Pictures were presented daily at 3pm and 8pm, and two years later, direct from the Picton Hall, Liverpool, the New Century Animated Picture Co. gave an exhibition of 10,000 pictures.

The Southport Opera House and Winter Gardens Co. took over the complex in 1905 and instituted the reconstruction of the Pavilion as the 1,200 seat Albert Hall Palace of Varieties. At first-floor level this was reached from the entrance hall by a broad staircase divided by a central iron balustrade leading up to the large lounge from which three entrances gave access to the left-hand side of the stalls. The balcony was entered in a similar position, a continuation of the stairway being ascended to the second-floor lounge. Extending along the side walls from the central section facing the stage, the front of the balcony was in the form of separate box fronts, each area containing four seats, and bounded by pairs of columns extending up to the cornice.

Above this the ceiling curved up to a great height featuring an abundance of carved plaster work, and from the former use as a concert hall, the oval windows were covered to prevent the admission of daylight. The orchestra pit fronted a 40ft. wide, arched proscenium behind which was a large stage and considerable dressing room accommodation.

The Albert Hall Palace of Varieties was opened by a lessee, Mr. Charles Parker, on 26th December 1905 with performances at 3pm and 7.30pm of the Great Caban with his marvellous performing ponies, donkeys and dogs, supported by a powerful company of star artistes. Admission at 6d, 1/- and 2/- were stated as popular prices. In 1906, the variety shows were followed at 10.15pm by the latest films on the Bioscope, which later became a daily afternoon attraction.

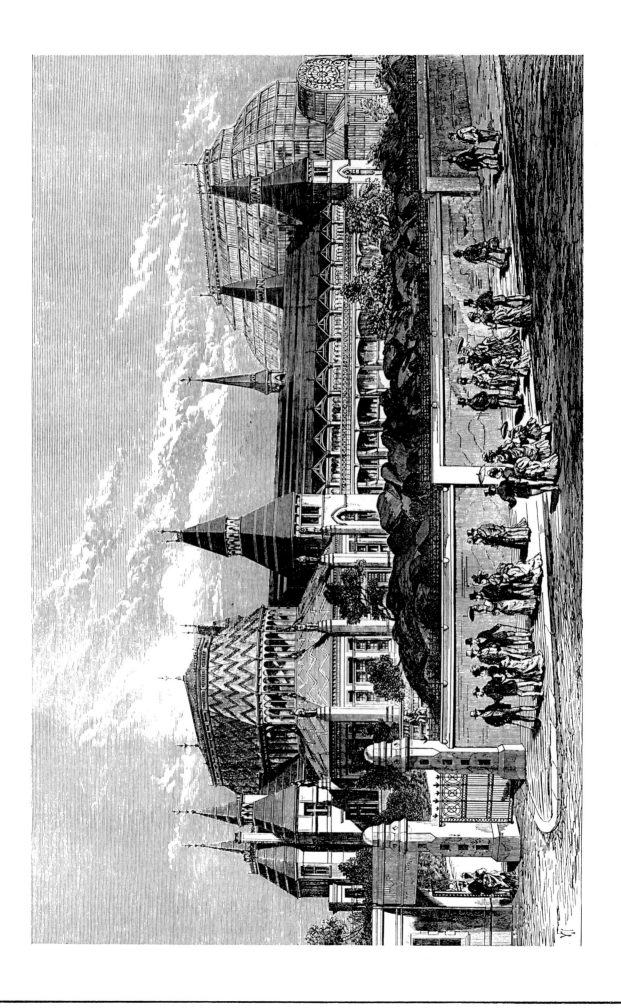

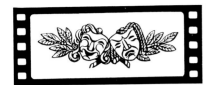

Mr. W. Simpson Cross, the brother of Alderman James Cross, a former Lord Mayor of Liverpool took over the lease of the theatre and adjoining parts of the complex c1910, styling himself as Director General, transferring his zoo park on Scarisbrick Road to the Winter Gardens. The theatre was then re-named the Empire, below which the aquarium was replaced by the Empire Zoodrome and a roller skating rink, of which, as general manager, Mr. William Walker was later to become one of the town's most successful cinema managers.

The Empire closed as a variety and picture theatre on 22 February 1913, and during the following two weeks the work of renovation, and re-decoration with a rich colour scheme in exquisite taste enhancing the architectural features, was stated to have transformed the hall into an attractive, luxurious and first class picture theatre. For this purpose the projection box was considerably enlarged to accommodate an additional machine; the directors of the new company, of which the chairman was Alderman Austin stating their intention to excel all previous film performances, which, for some time past on Sunday evenings had attracted far larger crowds than at other cinemas in the town.

Opposite: The Winter Gardens from the Promenade, showing the entrance gates to the ten acre site. The engraving was made the year the Winter Gardens opened, 1874.
Drawing: Geoff Wright

Right: The Winter Gardens from the Promenade with the Conservatory in the right foreground. The lower photo is taken from the Lord Street side with the Pavilion on the right. In 1891 the skating rink adjacent to Lord Street was demolished and replaced by the Opera House.
Photos: Geoff Wright

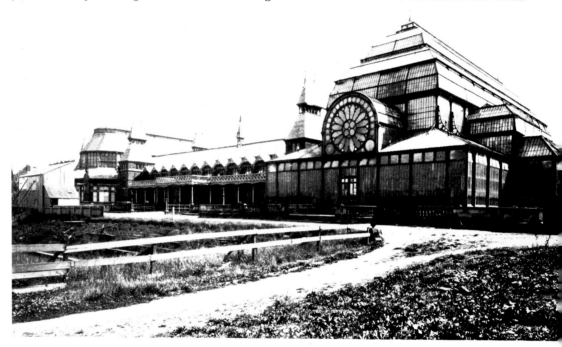

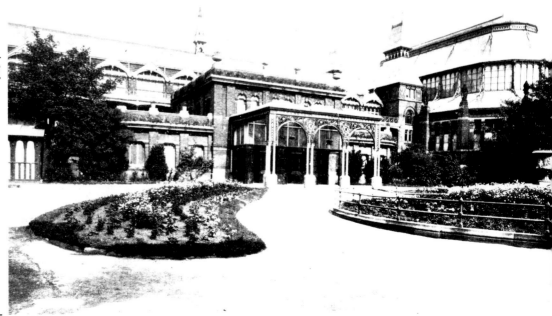

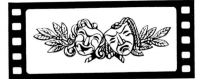

The Pavilion (1874-1905) as originally built. This later became the Empire and after improvements to provide greater comfort, the Empire Picture Theatre. It then became the West End and finally, the Scala.
Photo: Geoff Wright

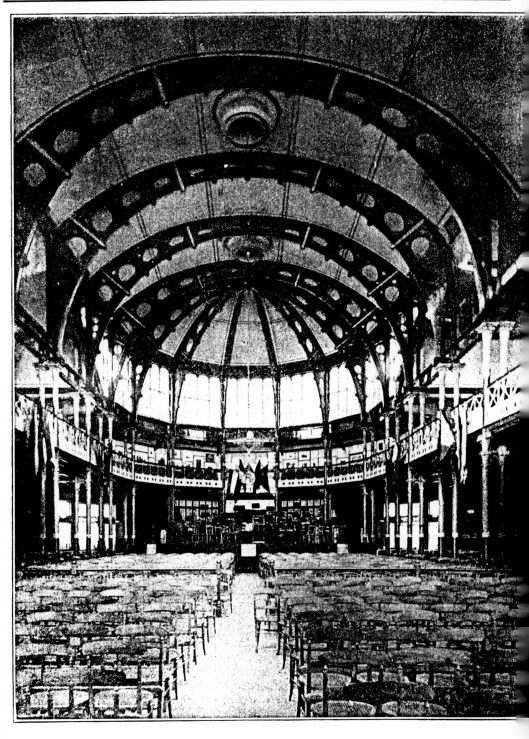

Despite the numerous entertainments in the town it was considered that the Empire should attain a premier position in popularity, for in addition to the internal comfort of the theatre, it had the advantage of direct access from the spacious Promenade Hall, which provided pleasant shelter for patrons waiting for the doors to open.

The Empire Picture Theatre opened on Monday 10 March 1913 with a packed house which included a large number of prominent townspeople, who were enthusiastic at the pleasing transformation of the hall and expressed satisfaction with the varied programme of films arranged by the new proprietors. The feature film was a drama entitled *When the Heart Speaks* and the supporting programme included *Why Jim Reformed, The Cringer* and *The Pony who paid the Rent*. For this and subsequent programmes, performances were at 3pm, 7pm and 9pm, also one performance on Sunday evenings at 8.15pm. Admission to the balcony was 1/- stalls 6d and pit stalls 2d, and afternoon tea was provided free of charge to patrons of the 6d and 1/- seats.

At this time, a complete break was made with the past with the closure of the zoo and the area in the basement replaced by the Empire Roller Rink which was opened on 7 April 1913.

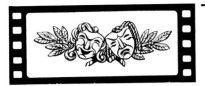

The Scala became the first "talkie" cinema in Southport with *The Singing Fool* in 1929.
Advert: *Southport Visitor*

In the early twenties, owned by Councillor F. Hayes, the Winter Gardens, styled as "The Home of Amusements" included The West End Cinema (formerly the Empire), The West End Cafe, a ballroom, aviary and aquarium. In September 1921 it was announced that Councillor Hayes had entered into an agreement with Alfred Levy, known in trade circles as "the film king", to take over the running of the cinema, which he promptly re-named the Scala. The object was to link up his name with that of his successful cinemas in Birmingham and Liverpool. Film bookings by the Levy circuit commenced on 5 September 1921 with *Mystery of the Wakeford Case* and *Weavers of Life*, daily at 3pm, 6.45 and 8.45pm with admission prices, 6d, Is 2d and Is 7d.

Under Alfred Levy's control the Scala was the first "talkie" cinema in Southport, Western Electric sound system at a cost of £4,000 being installed for the Grand Opening on 22 April 1929 of *The Singing Fool* starring Al Jolson. Large crowds attended, paying increased prices of 1/-, 2/- and 3/- for the performances at 3pm, 6.40pm and 8.50pm. Alfred Levy relinquished control of the Scala early in 1930 when a private company, Scala Southport Ltd was formed to acquire the cinema and billiard hall, with booking of films continued by the Southport Winter Gardens Ltd.

First in Southport with the "talkies" the Scala was also first with the latest in pictures - The Wide Screen, the only one of its kind to be seen outside of London. This attraction commenced on 21 July 1930 with George Arliss as *Disraeli* to which at the bargain matinees there were 1,200 seats at 6d.

By this time, the Scala was a separate building with entrance and bar extending partly across the new thoroughfare, Kingsway, linking Lord Street with the promenade and opened in June 1930. This was constructed through the site of the Winter Gardens Promenade Hall, demolished shortly after the destruction by fire of the Opera House in December 1929, which led to the demolition of the Winter Gardens complex by stages until 1933.

In order to completely clear Kingsway, it was necessary to take down the Scala entrance and bar, and in July 1930 plans were submitted to the town council for a new splayed frontage with an entrance at either end and a centre portion incorporating a large advertising site. This was shortly afterwards constructed of Portland stone relieved by horizontal bands of brick with entrances at either end surmounted by a canopy. Above, the three tall, arched windows of the first-floor lounge were set behind an architectural feature incorporating arches supported by columns. The entrances gave access at either end of the new foyer adjacent to Kingsway with the pay-box opposite the entrance facing Lord Street. Beyond the pay-box a short flight of stairs rose to the original foyer to which there was direct access by a stairway from the side elevation where entrance/exit doors were set between columns supporting a stonework architectural feature including the cinema name in large letters above a streamer poster frame.

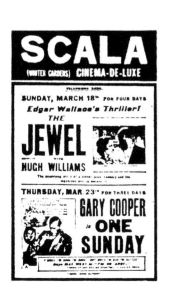

13

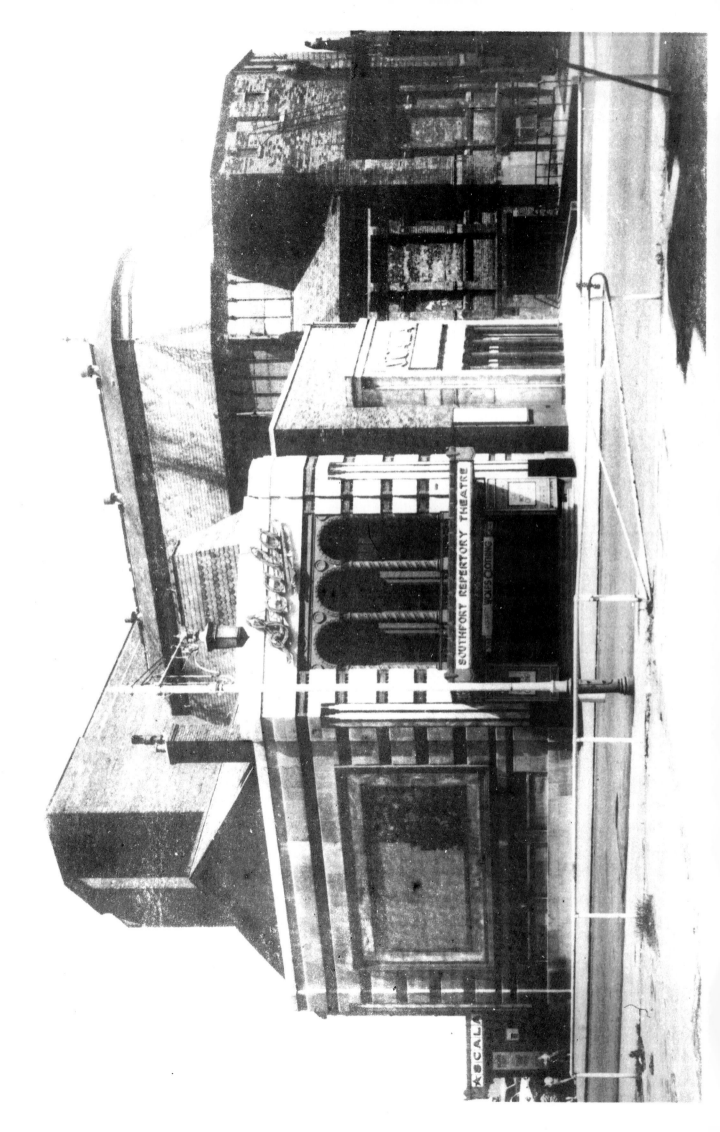

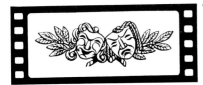

In the mid thirties the Scala was taken over by a newly formed company, Associated Southport Cinemas whose general manager was Mr.W.Peel Smith, formerly chief supervisor of the General Theatre Corporation. The extensive interior of the Scala building provided adequate space for the company offices, from which they also controlled the Palace, Lord Street, Coliseum, Nevill Street and the Plaza, Ainsdale, also for a short time from 1938, the Trocadero and Forum, Lord Street.

The Scala was closed on 20 November 1938 for modernisation and re-seating which reduced the capacity to 1,043 and in the centre of the balcony the separate boxes were replaced by a straight front.

Re-opening on Christmas Day 1938 with Walt Disney's *Snow White and the Seven Dwarfs* , the Scala was open as a cinema until 18 February 1939, then beginning another period of closure for the re-building of the stage block to provide a 34ft. deep stage. Opening as a 'live' theatre on Easter Monday 1939, Ernest Binn's *Arcadian Follies* ran until the outbreak of war on 3rd Sept. 1939. After a period of cine-variety, the follies returned for the 1940 summer season until 14th September, after which, with the exception of musical programmes by Bill Gregson and his Broadcasting Band at 3pm on Sundays, the Scala screened films, ending with *Yellow Sky* featuring Gregory Peck on 4 October 1953.

The Scala then became the home of the Southport Repertory Co. who commenced their winter season on 6 October 1953 with the play *Lady Frederick* and continued with their productions until the theatre finally closed on 20 January 1962. Four months later demolition of the building had been completed, removing the last unit of the Winter Gardens complex and leaving only the terrace of that name and Pavilion Buildings on Coronation Walk as a reminder of the great Victorian enterprise of Southport's golden age.

The only use made of the Scala site has been as a large car park.

Opposite and below: Apart from the roof, very little remains of the original Winter Gardens Pavilion in these two photos. A comparison with the photo at the bottom of page 11 shows how much times have changed. A supermarket car park now occupies the site while the supermarket itself is on Lord Street in front of the site.
Photos: Mike Yelland (opposite) and W.E. Marsden (below)

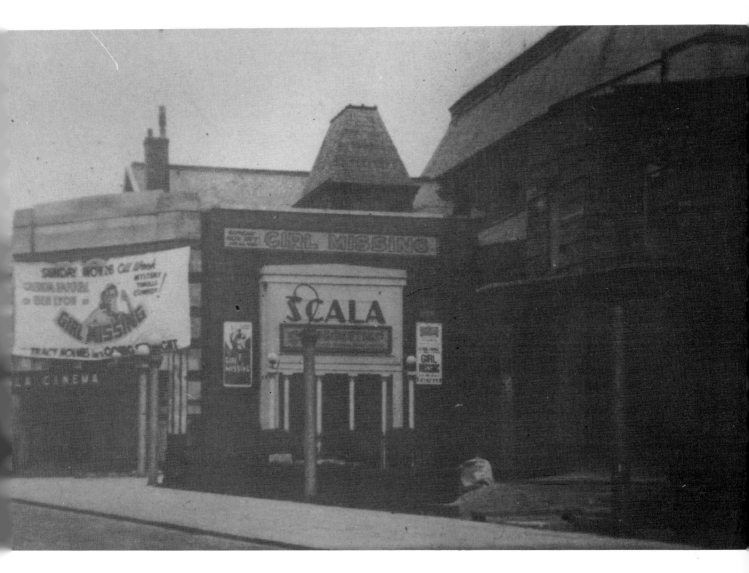

15

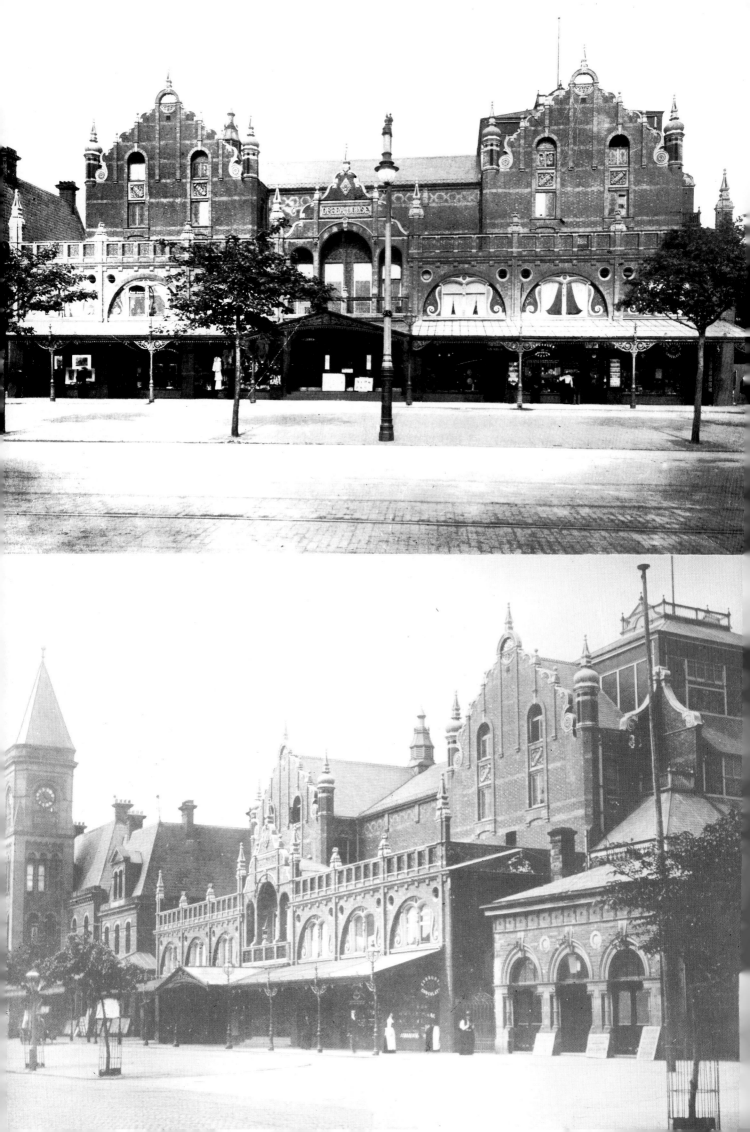

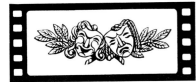

The Opera House, the most sumptuous building in the Winter Gardens complex, was opened in 1891 and destroyed by fire in 1929. Considered one of Frank Matcham's masterpieces, the Opera House was built on a site previously occupied by a skating rink and afterwards, a dance hall. The entrance to the Empire (the former Pavilion) and then the Scala, can be seen to the right of the Opera House. This entrance was demolished and a new frontage of cream tiles built on the side of the Scala when Kingsway was built. The building on the left with the clock tower was Lord Street railway station. After closure it became the Ribble bus station and is now incorporated in the Winter Gardens Shopping Centre.
Photos: Geoff Wright

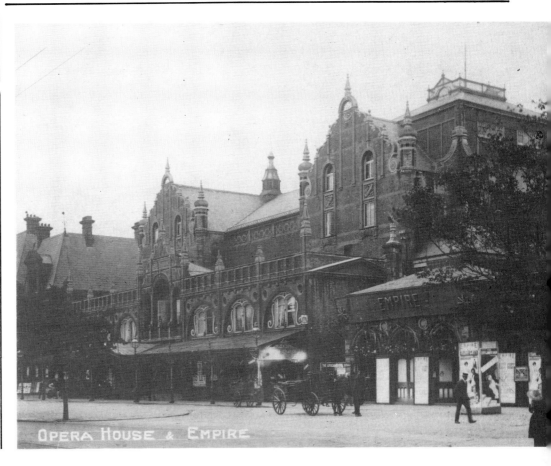

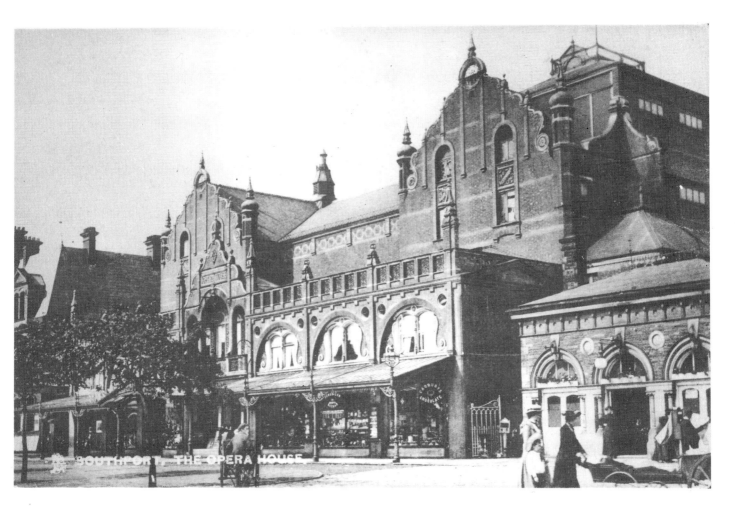

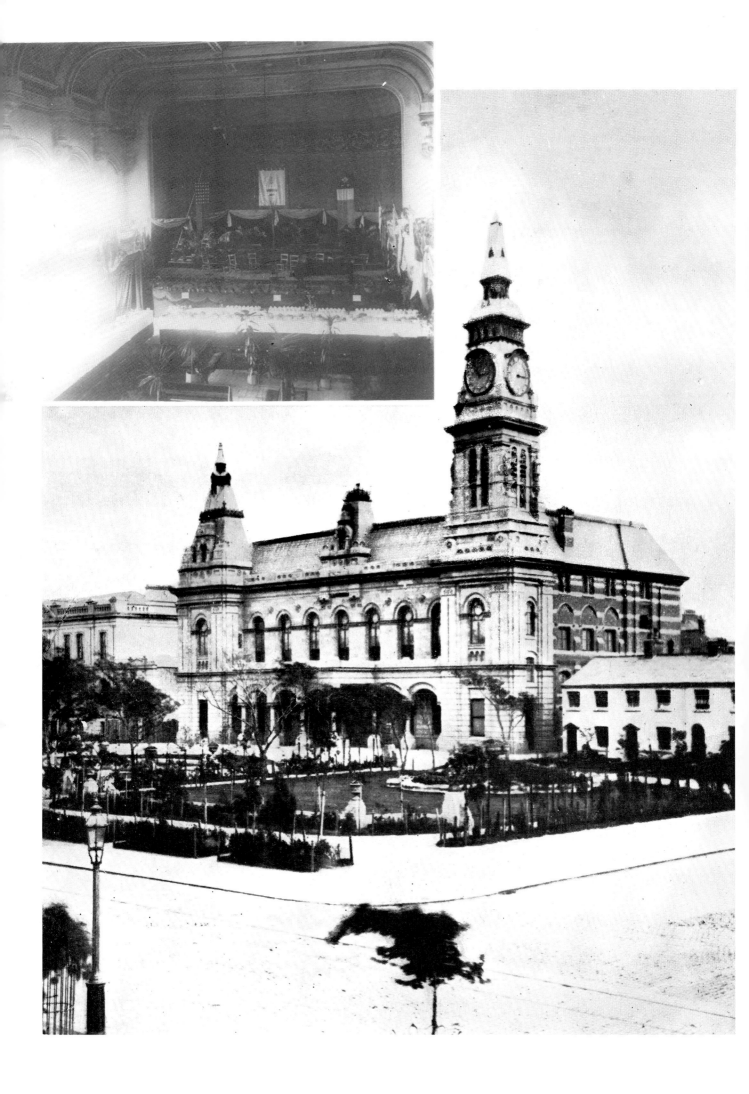

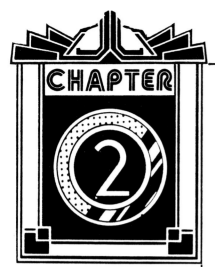

CHAPTER 2

The Cambridge Hall was designed by Maxwell & Tuke. The elegant tower at the corner is but a minor landmark compared to their later work. Maxwell & Tuke went on to design Blackpool Tower, opened 1894, and New Brighton Tower, opened 1900.
Photo: Geoff Wright

The interior (inset) shows the hall arranged for dinner or buffet.
Photo: Metropolitan Borough of Sefton

THE CAMBRIDGE HALL/ARTS CENTRE, Lord Street, Southport

This magnificent building adjacent to the Atkinson Library was designed by Messrs Maxwell & Tuke of Bury, Greater Manchester, and erected in 1874 by Messrs Haywards of Southport at a cost of £30,000. The foundation stone was laid on 9 October 1872 by the Princess Mary of Cambridge, from whom the original name of the hall was derived, and it was the enterprise of the Southport Corporation as a venue for public meetings, concerts and banquets. Despite considerable internal re-construction in 1974, the original imposing facade remains after 115 years. Constructed entirely of stone, an arcade extends along the greater part of the frontage at ground level, from which in the centre projects a massive carriage port with three archways supported by columns in matching style to those of the arcade. At first-floor level there is a line of tall windows, and above the carriage port, a balcony from which there was originally a fine view of the coastline. At the south front corner a commanding feature is the elegant tower with illuminated clocks, once with chimes, the gift of Mr. Atkinson of Free Library fame.

In the centre of the arcade the entrance doors lead into a vestibule which extends into the centre of the spacious foyer, with at each side, areas allocated for offices, assembly and store rooms, and although this original plan has undergone considerable alteration, there still remains the large stone fireplace upon which is carved the year of the building's erection - 1874. The impressive architecture of the period features a series of three archways across the foyer supported by short marble columns with floriated capitals. These are mounted upon tall bases each supporting a square architrave at the base of the archways, above which the high ceiling is deeply coffered and divided into separate areas with carved cornices. Opposite the main entrance at the far end of the foyer, described as the grand staircase, this has a carved stone balustrade at the left hand side and is divided in the centre by an iron balustrade supporting two hand-rails. Extending to the left, the stairway has an attractive background of high, arched-topped stained-glass windows, whilst at the left-hand side, white marble statues hold above torch-style light-fittings. At the head of the staircase, doors at the right of a wide landing give access to the right-hand side of the auditorium, and originally stairways led up to the balcony.

Occupying the entire length of the building on the first floor, the auditorium is 120ft. in length, 50ft wide and 37ft. high. This originally had a flat lower floor which could be used for dances and various functions, whilst extending along either side and across the rear, a panelled-fronted balcony was supported by columns. Decoration of the side walls is by large panels, the tops of which are curved, and above these from the cornice, the ceiling curves up to the straight central span. At the front of the hall, a proscenium formerly divided it from the full-width stage to which there was access by a short flight of stairs at either side. It is recorded that the Cambridge Hall in 1874 had capacity for nearly 2,000 people and seating for 1,500, but it is noteworthy that since re-construction in 1974, the seating capacity has been below 500.

The Grand Gala opening took place on 6th October 1874, when the ceremony was performed by the Right Honourable R.A. Cross, M.P., an occasion which was marked by public rejoicing with a Grand Procession and a Public Banquet for which music was provided by military and orchestral bands. The first stage performance was during the latter half of the week from Thursday, 8th October when it was announced that the stage was elegantly decorated for the appearance of F.J. Cooper's Great American Aggregation Company's "The Female Christys", twelve unrivalled artistes representing a great bevy of beauty, each chosen and trained for a speciality. For the performance at 8pm, seats could be reserved for 3/- whilst admission to the balcony was 2/- with rear seats at 1/- and rear balcony 6d.

For almost 100 years the Cambridge Hall was a favourite venue for lectures, concerts and various types of theatrical performances, but in later years becoming very shabby and suffered a decline before its centenary. In 1972 with the support of the Arts Council, a scheme was inaugurated by Southport Corporation for the internal reconstruction and refurbishment of the Grade II listed building. Architects, civil and services engineers and quantity surveyors were appointed by the Building Design Partnership, Preston, for the major scheme, which in 1974 was completed at a cost of £175,000 to provide a re-styled 496 seat auditorium, committee rooms, a licensed bar and exhibition areas. The principal item was the re-construction of the auditorium, in which the balcony was dispensed with in favour of a stepped flooring from front to rear with a separate section of front stalls seats separated from those of the centre and rear by a crossover gangway, from which, due to the higher level of the new floor, short stairways led down to the main entrance/exit door to the first-floor landing. Towards the rear the increased height of the floor provided space below for a mezzanine floor, allocated for a licensed bar and refreshment room.

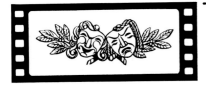

The stage was extended forward with a splayed front, to which the seating at about the same level was arranged accordingly in three sections across the hall with centre and side blocks. In the absence of footlights the stage was illuminated by spotlights and semi-concealed lighting in the roof void. Since it was the intention to use the hall also as a cinema, a full sized masked screen could be lowered into position on the stage, and a projection suite was constructed in the area of the former rear balcony. These facilities were added to provide a superior venue for the Southport Film Guild, who had won the Film Society of the Year Award in 1969 and had used this to assist the campaign for an Arts Centre.

On the ground floor the new plans provided for new ticket and advance booking offices to the right of the entrance, and at the far end, a coffee bar in the area comfortably furnished as a lounge. Separated by metal-framed doors, the vestibule led into the re-styled foyer in which, contrasting with the old architectural features, there was a strong, modern decorative treatment in red, and floor covering of yellow and black striped carpet.

The building was re-opened by the Metropolitan Borough of Sefton as the Arts Centre on 21 September 1974 when the distinction of providing the first entertainment went to the Southport Music Festival, which was appropriate since the hall had been its venue since 1949. This was followed by leading musical and theatrical events, but links with the Victorian past (as the Cambridge Hall) were recalled on 6 October 1974 when the 100th Anniversary was marked by a Victorian evening of music and song to which the audience was invited to attend in Victorian costume. On 15 October, the Southport Film Guild with greatly increased membership, presented the first of their film performances at the Arts Centre, and since that time, advertised as "Cinema at the Centre" films have been a regular attraction on dates not allocated to 'live' entertainment.

In November 1987 another major restoration and redecoration scheme was commenced, due to which the Arts Centre was closed during the period 16 January to 28 February inclusive. The effects are most impressive and in a style more appropriate to that of the original architecture. On entering, it is first observed that attractive glass-panelled wooden doors replace the former metal-framed type, and the second set of doors have been dispensed with, allowing from the vestibule a more open aspect of the entrance hall. Therein the ticket booking office has been re-sited on the left-hand side adjacent to the

The Cambridge Hall (on the left) was joined by the Atkinson Free Library and the Town Hall. Both buildings are still an attractive feature of Lord Street.
Picture: Geoff Wright

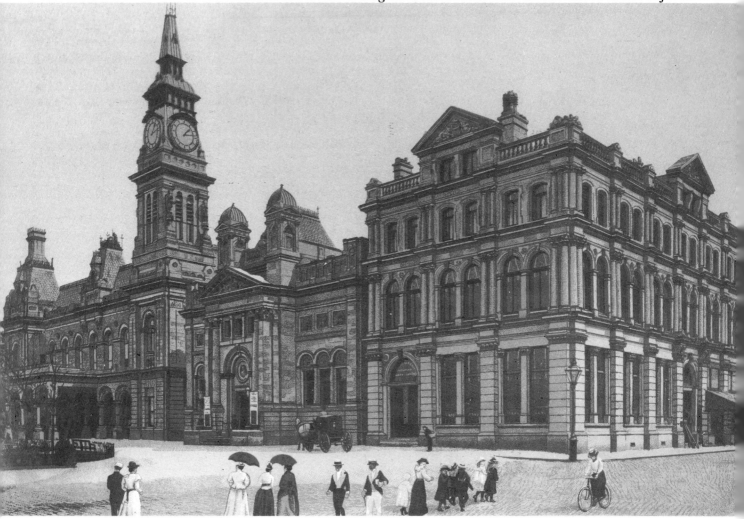

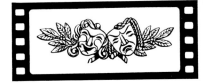

fireplace and the right-hand side allocated as a display area, whilst the refreshment bar has been removed, no doubt by reason of this facility being provided on the first floor. The predominant strong red of the previous decorations has been replaced by the more subdued colour of damask rose with plaster mouldings of the side walls and the archways relieved by blue and gold, above which the separate corniced areas of the ceiling are in deep blue. The colour treatment of the columns is dark brown veined with white, and above, mounted upon the architraves, are shaded electric fittings from which light is cast on the archways. The entire scheme is complemented by the new floor covering of patterned carpet with background of dark blue.

The Arts Centre was re-opened on 28 February 1989 when at 7.45pm the Southport Film Guild presented the film *Salvador* (USA 1986) to members and guests only, whilst the remainder of the week was devoted to 'live' entertainment.

The entire scheme of refurbishment was completed in the autumn of 1989, when, 15 years after its first centenary, the question of possible survival to a second must surely come to mind.

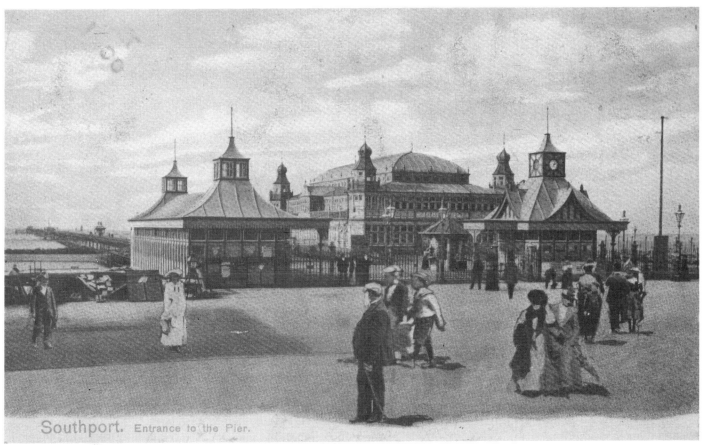

Southport. Entrance to the Pier.

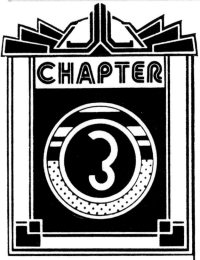

Above: The Pier Pavilion
Photo: Geoff Wright

PIER PAVILION, Promenade, Southport

The new theatre was part of a large scheme of improvements, including the widening of the pier, commenced in 1901 following the destruction by fire of the old Pavilion four years previously. The plans of the architect, Mr. R. Knill-Freeman, FRIBA, provided for the setting back of the new theatre from the promenade by about 60ft to allow space for a large forecourt sectioned off from the promenade and with toll offices where pedestrians were to pay for admission to the pier, which extended from the left-hand side of the theatre. At a total cost of about £14,000 an important part of the scheme was the vastly superior theatre, with exterior surrounded by spacious balconies affording pleasant views of the sea front, the promenade and the lake at either side, which it was anticipated would prove a great attraction during the summer months. The shell of the building was formed of steel and cast iron filled in with panelling and moulded framing of the lower part and glass in the upper with ornamental heads, whilst the main roof was finished with an ornamental iron railing and a weather vane at each end. An octagonal turret surmounted by a cupola and ornamental iron finial adorned the upper part of the four corners of the building, and it was divided from the pier by iron railings with electric light standards spaced along.

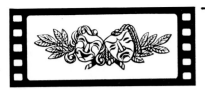

In the centre of the frontage the principal entrance gave access to the Pavilion via a pair of swing doors on each side of the ticket office, beyond which were the entrances to the stalls floor and stairways to the gallery. The auditorium, 90ft long and 53ft wide had recessed alcoves on each side, galleries on three sides, and a seating capacity of about 1,500 but including the standing room in the spacious promenade behind the rear rows of the galleries it was estimated that the hall would hold about 2,000 people. At either side of the well-elevated stage were connecting dressing rooms, and an emergency exit and stairway from the gallery. The gallery front, the proscenium and a portion of the ceiling were specially designed and finished in enriched fibrous plaster. The building was lit throughout by electric light but in case of emergency a small system of gas light was installed and heating was by gas stoves.

Under the ownership of the Southport Pier Co. Ltd., and the management of Mr. W. H. Scott, the inaugural opening of the new Pavilion by Alderman T.P. Griffiths, J.P. on New Year's Day 1902 was reported as an undoubted success despite the wet weather. All the public and representative men in the town with their wives were invited to the afternoon proceedings when the ceremonial was all conducted from the stage. In the evening, the Grand Concert at 7.30pm, for the first public entertainment the Pavilion was crowded by 1,800 people for whom admission was - front seats 2/-, second seats 1/- and balcony 6d.

Brass band and orchestral concerts formed the entertainment until 1906 when the theatre was leased to a Mr. Sam Berry for variety entertainments, and in 1908 the lessees, the MacNagthen Vaudeville circuit opened with similar entertainment on 11 May (Whit Monday) when the bill included "Raymond's Bio-Tableaux", Matt Raymond's silent Pictures in the once nightly performance at 8pm.

In 1910 a sort of early *Opportunity Knocks* was held at trial matinees to discover talent and any worthwhile acts were given a tour of the MacNagthen circuit, then comprising about a dozen variety theatres countrywide.

Silent pictures returned in 1913, presumably in an attempt to compete with the four cinemas by that time open in the town. But the Pavilion was principally a "Live" theatre, which during its 70 years was a mecca for those who enjoyed the best in light entertainment, although serious drama and Shakespearian plays were also presented. The list of distinguished artistes who appeared is extremely lengthy and includes Gracie Fields, George Formby, senior and junior, Charlie Chaplin, also George Robey, and it was at the Pavilion that Flanagan and Allen first sang *Underneath the Arches*.

In 1931 a scheme of alterations and decorations was carried out, and to enable this to be completed, the theatre was closed during the week commencing 16 February. It was reported that in addition to the considerable improvements the decorations were charming throughout in colours of pink, cream and gold, and the stage and boxes re-curtained in warm red plush, whilst the floors, luxuriously re-carpeted had transformed the place into one of the most attractive entertainment houses in the town.

The theatre was reopened by the Mayor of Southport, Councillor Alfred Peploe, O.B.E. on 23rd February 1931 when a season of West End plays was inaugurated. Described as "High Class but not High Brow", these were presented by the eminent and distinguished actor, Henry Baynton and his famous repertory players, commencing with Israel Zampwill's famous drama *The Melting Pot* for which the theatre was crowded for the performance at 7.30pm.

This was among the locations used for a short time by the Southport Dramatic Club before acquiring their permanent home at the Little Theatre. At the Pavilion the first of a short season of plays commenced on 16 March 1931 and was followed by other productions of the S.D.C. until November of that year. The Pavilion remained under the ownership of the Southport Pier Co.until 1936 when it was purchased by the corporation who renamed it the Casino and continued to present the best in light entertainment until 1963 when it was leased to the Southport Repertory Co. for stage plays following the company's nine years at the Scala, which terminated when the theatre was closed for demolition in January 1962. But only seven years later, in 1970, this was also the fate of the Casino, the building having been condemned by the council. The site was re-developed with the present amusement arcade known as Funland.

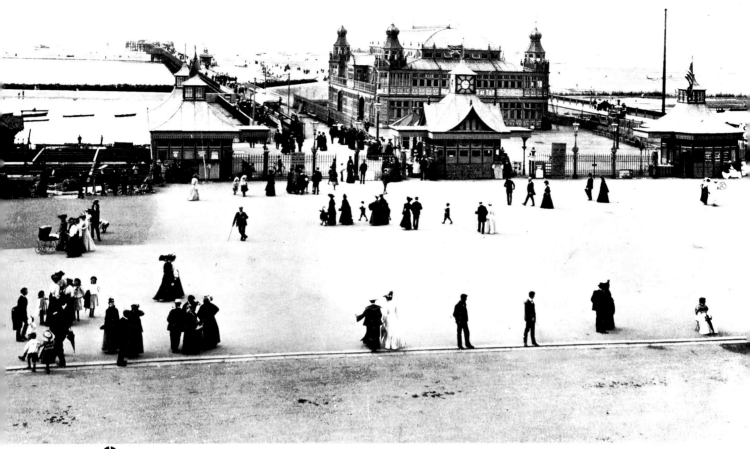

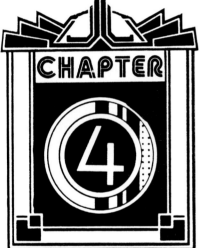

CHAPTER 4

The elevation of Southport's first purpose-built cinema. Originally the Picturedrome, it became the Forum in 1933.
Elevation: Janet Jenkins

PICTUREDROME/FORUM, Lord Street, Southport.

The building of Southport's first purpose-built cinema was commenced in February 1910 and completed in only 13 weeks for the opening on 9th May. To the design of Southport architects, Campbell & Fairhurst, it was considered to be a model of what the picture theatre of the future was to be, and the architects were congratulated upon having designed an architecturally superior building in keeping with the environment, with the attractive white frontage being enhanced by the land in front laid out in the form of an ornamental garden by Southport Corporation.

The building, with regard to height and general outline, was regulated entirely by the owner of the valuable site with a view to keeping within the law regarding the right of light, to comply with which, the building was kept down to the legal limit.

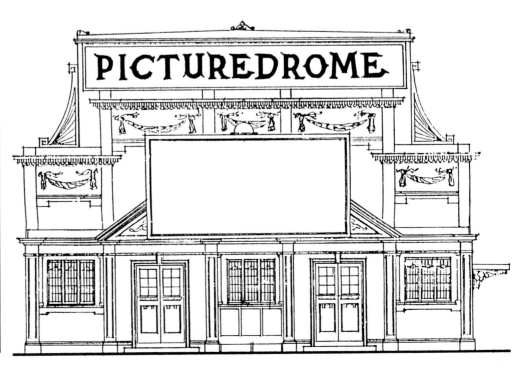

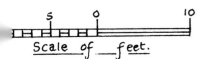

Scale of feet.

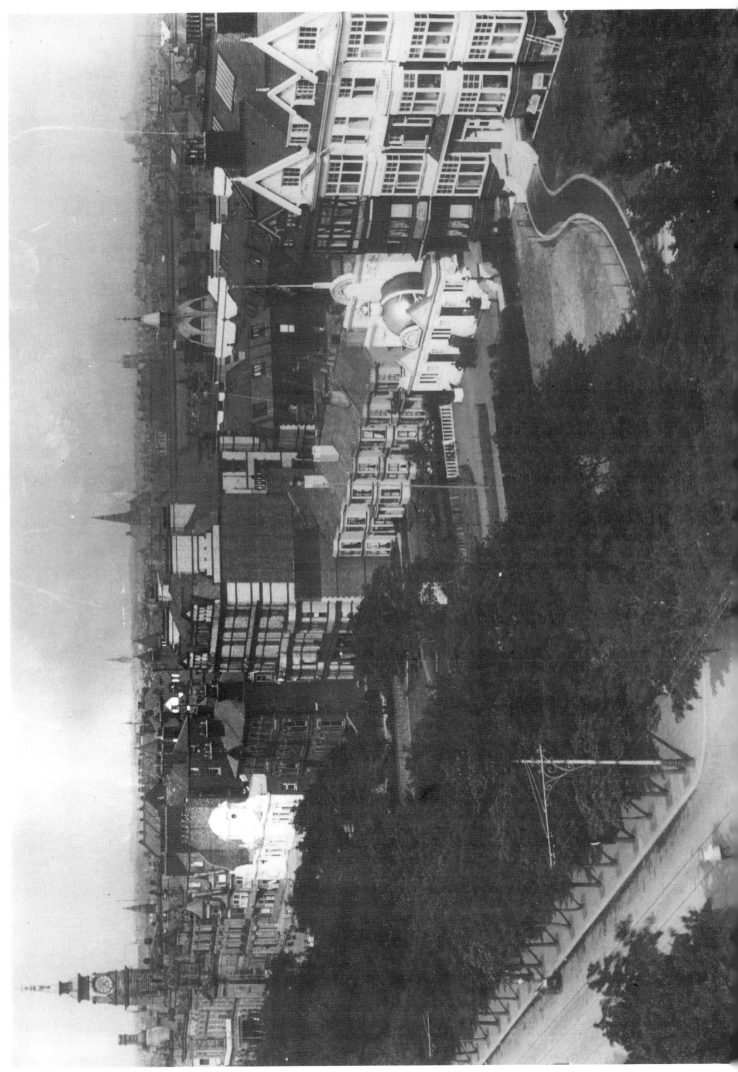

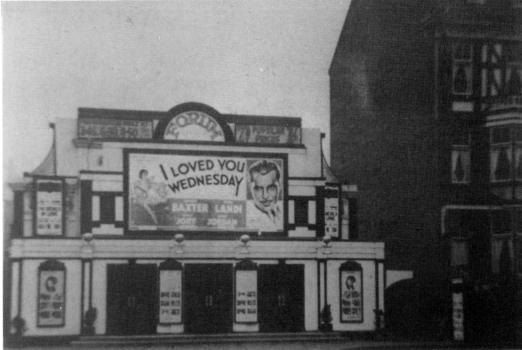

Although small compared to the cinemas of later years, the frontage was ornate with attractive carved designs on the facing of white painted cement. The lower part was built forward of the main structure with, in the centre of the roof, a large dome and mounted upon this was a small dome supported by columns. This elevation included two separate entrance ways and three windows which were flanked by pilasters whilst elaborately-carved pediments surmounted the entrances. The double doors of these had attractive glass and wood panels, and gave access to the entrance hall with floor of mosaic, and above a dado of maroon. The white painted walls had panels in pale green.

The upper part of the frontage was constructed on two levels with the taller, principal centre flanked by small sections at a lower level. These were bounded by pilasters, of which two in the centre extended up to an attractive arch and from the base of this, the coping extended to the sides. This method of construction effectively screened from view the auditorium roof when observing the frontage from a position directly opposite.

The building consisted of a steel frame filled in with breeze blocks, plastered on the inside and cemented on the outside. The floor was laid solid upon breeze concrete, the ceiling was of fibrous plaster and the slates of compressed asbestos. As the woodwork was confined almost solely to the floor and doors, the building was claimed to be as near to fireproof as possible.

The Picturedrome was among the first buildings in the country designed for animated pictures, and complying with the Cinematograph Act of 1909, which for the safety of the public regulated that the projection room should be completely cut off from the auditorium. In this case entrance was by means of a spiral staircase from the entrance hall to a flat roof from which there was access to the projection room, sited within the domed area of the front elevation. The only connection with the auditorium consisted of two small, square, steel-shuttered windows, through which passed the rays of light from the projectors. The stadium-style auditorium had a seating capacity of approximately 700, and more than adequate to comply with the act, eight exits were provided and above each double door, electrically illuminated boxes displayed the word EXIT. Except for the front stalls where forms were fitted, each patron had a tip-up seat, all on a raked floor covered by a handsome Axminster carpet, which rose 4ft from the stage to the rear, facilitating the view of the screen. This was about 14ft square and formed on the solid wall at the rear of the stage. It was treated with special paint and four coats of plaster, each laid on in a different direction.

In addition to its main purpose as a cinema, the possibility of concerts was also provided for with dressing rooms at either side of the stage.

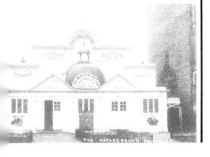

The scheme of decoration was described as most attractive with the walls and barrel-shaped ceiling painted white with a dado of maroon. Red plush curtains covered the windows and doors, and there were red silk shades over the electric globes which lit the hall, making it possible for patrons to see all parts during performances.

"THE WORLD IN MOTION."

The PICTUREDROME

Southport's Beautiful Picture House.

EASILY FIRST !   ALWAYS THE LATEST PICTURES !

COOL IN SUMMER—WARM IN WINTER—THAT IS THE TEMPERATURE !

Sunday Evening, Sept 21st, at 8-15.   A Powerful Photo Play entitled—

"THE GANTON MYSTERY."

and Specially Selected High-class Programme.

Monday, Tuesday and Wednesday
SEPT. 22nd, 23rd, and 24th.

Exclusive—The Great American Society Drama, in Three Parts. Entitled—

"THE IMPOSTOR."

Along the Italian Coast

A beautiful and interesting series showing the various beauty spots along the coast of Italy, distinguished by remarkably clear photography and excellent light effects.

That the Italian coast, along the Gulf of Genoa, possesses many scenes well worthy of being perpetuated in moving pictures, is amply shown in this splendid subject. Views of Oneglia, Port Mausizio, Poggio Arma and St. Eleene, San Remo with its brilliant little harbour, and many other delightful pleasure haunts are shown in rapid succession, showing scenes of beauty difficult to realise without being witnessed. All the scenes are tinted and coloured and are real objects of admiration.

A Box of Canine Mischief

A box is delivered to Mr. Carl Bonner, together with a note announcing the arrival of a present. When the box is opened a smart little terrier jumps out, but Carl dislikes dogs and chases him off, only to find him begging at his side the next moment. Carl goes to a café, where a careless waiter spills soup on him ; the little dog turns up and runs for a cloth to repair the damage. This pleases Carl, and he allows his new pet to go for a walk with him. He soon regrets it, however, as the dog gets him into endless scrapes, and when he at length reaches home he sends for the box, packs up his canine present and scrawls "unknown" across the address. The box immediately jumps off the table, trots through the gate away to the station. where it boards a train and is carried away. to the joy of its late owner.

A Popular Song on the Vivaphone, &c.

Thursday, Friday, & Saturday,
SEPT. 25th, 26th, and 27th.

Exclusive—A Stirring Drama full of Human Interest, entitled—

" Her Supreme Sacrifice "

in Three Parts, in which a woman sacrifices wealth and social position to devote her life to the man she loved.

Lakes of Bois de Boulogne
Polidor's Silver Crown
Murphy's I.O.U.
Making the Luneville Delftware

A particularly interesting and instructive industrial film, showing the whole process most minutely and in an entertaining manner.

ORDER OF PICTURES.

Mixing the soft clay which is brought from Champagne.
Rolling out the earthenware.
Moulding plates and dishes.
The pieces are now put into frames to undergo a first firing process.
Putting in and sealing up the ovens.
After baking for 24 hours at a heat of 1800 degrees, the ovens are opened and the batch removed.
Throwing out the imperfect pieces.
The printing rooms.
Enamelling the ware.
A collection of beautiful Delftware.

A Popular Song on the Vivaphone
Gaumont Graphic of Daily Happenings
&c., &c.

 Have your Afternoon Tea at the Picturedrome, it is served Free in the 1s. and 6d. Seats, at about 3-30. We only use the best of everything. THOM'S TEA, WOODHEAD'S CREAM, and HUNTLEY and PALMER'S BISCUITS.

AFTERNOON PERFORMANCE Commences at 3-0. Doors open 2-45.
EVENING PERFORMANCES Commence at 7 & 9. Doors open 6-45 & 8-50.
SUNDAY EVENING PERFORMANCE Commences at 8-15. Doors open at 7-55.

PRICES: 1S., 6D., & 3D.

Children Half-price at Matinees to 1s. and 6d. Seats.

Stall Seats Booked and Reserved in advance. No extra Charge. TELEPHONE 19.
Picturedrome Box Office open Daily 10 a.m. to 10 p.m.

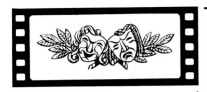

The proprietors, Southport Picturedrome Ltd., were a company financed by Manchester businessmen, who were interested in similar ventures in other parts of the country, but in connection with management and the supply of cinematograph films, the cinema opened under the control of the then expanding film exhibitor and later, renters. the Weisker Brothers.

The Grand Opening of the Picturedrome was arranged to take place on Saturday, 7th May 1910, and a great many invitations for the performance were issued by the directors,but owing to the death of King Edward VII, the opening was postponed until Monday, 9th May, and the invitations made available for any afternoon performance during that week. The entertainment advertised as "The World In Motion" comprised a varied and up-to-date series of pictures including the scenes outside the Palace before and after the death of the King. Large crowds attended the opening performances of films entitled - *Late the Shadow, All's Well That Ends Well, Where Teak Wood Grows, Why Girls Leave Home, The Pineapple Industry, The House Under Repair* and *Story of Circus Life*. The company announced that there would be three performances daily at 3pm, 7pm and 9pm, with the exception of Sunday when one performance with appropriate pictures would be shown at 8.15pm, and three changes of programme weekly on Sunday, Monday and Thursday. Admission prices were 1/-, 6d and 3d and children were admitted half price to the matinees in the 1/- and 6d seats, when tea was served free of charge. Patrons could book their seats in advance without extra charge at the box office open daily 10am to 10pm.

Stephenson's Guide to Southport of 1913 described the Picturedrome as an exceedingly comfortable place of entertainment, stating that the management from the first had shown unquestionable enterprise in obtaining all the latest pictures, which were entertaining, exciting and instructive.

The first Chaplin films seen in Southport were at the Picturedrome, and with piano accompaniment; famous films included *Quo Vadis?, Les Miserables,Lorna Doone* and *The Lady of the Camelias* starring the famous actress Sarah Bernhardt. Topical items included the Coronation of King George V, which was shown the same night, and there was a local newsreel photographed by the chief operator showing Lord Street shoppers every Saturday morning. Patrons enjoyed picking out familiar faces and commenting on ladies fashions!

Although the last cinema in the town to be converted for the "talkies", sound reproducing equipment known as the "Vivaphone" was presented as early as 1917. This was Hepworth's British sound-on-disc system, one of several at that time, and on 26th February 1929 it was re-introduced at the Picturedrome for the showing of the Universal picture *Lonesome* featuring Glenn Tryon and Barbara Kent. Patrons were asked to come and hear for themselves how favourably it compared with the more up-to-date systems of the (then) present day.

Thereafter, silent films continued until 7 February 1931 when the cinema was closed for one week for the installation of the latest Western Electric sound system and a new screen at a cost of £4,500. The re-opening as a "talkie" theatre was on Saturday, 14th February with the feature film *The Green Goddess* featuring George Arliss, followed on Monday by a 3 day showing of *Under the Greenwood Tree*. The cinema's advertisements stated - "To see it is to hear it, and to hear it is to be amazed" later changed to - "Our talkies are the Talk of The Town."

Little more than two years later, on 23rd April 1933, the final performance as the Picturedrome was with the film *Soldiers of Fortune* starring Jack Holt and Ralph Graves, also a Laurel & Hardy comedy.

The hall was closed for almost a month for modernisation and extensive alterations by a Southport architect, Mr G.E. Salt, which included considerable alteration of the frontage. At ground level, the two entrances and pediments were replaced by three pairs of doors, the windows were dispensed with and the intervening spaces occupied by stills frames. The dome above was removed for the construction of a larger projection room of which the rear wall was level with the lower part of the elevation. The large surface above the entrance doors was mostly covered by a large framed board used for a poster to advertise the current feature film, but in later years this was painted over with the cinema name Forum in gold letters and performance times. Other additions were four spotlights in pairs to illuminate the frontage and the provision of a canopy along the right-hand side of the building to shelter queueing patrons.

The architect's drawing of the
Picturedrome. A comparison with
the photo on page 24 will show how
closely the cinema was built to the
architect's original idea. The
drawing below shows the
auditorium when reconstructed as
the Forum in 1933.
Drawings: *Southport Visitor* (top)
and Pat McGowan (below).

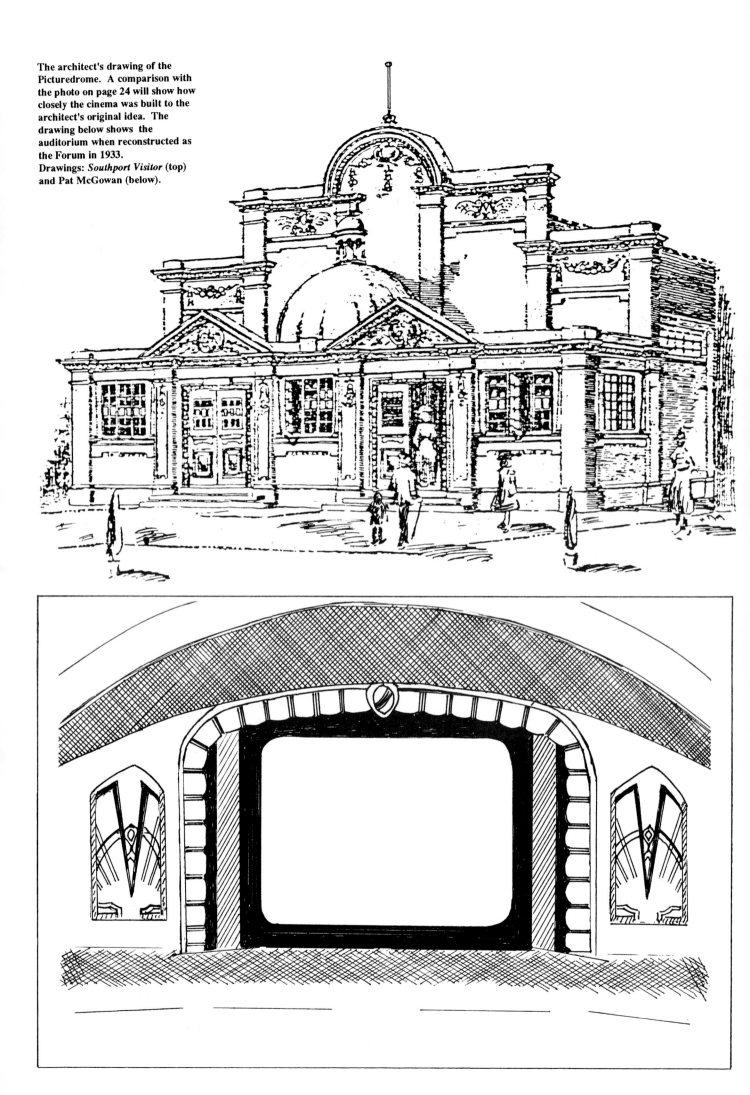

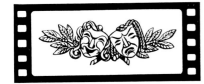

Internally, the foyer was re-styled in colours of silver and gold with the new pay-box and the doors in black and chromium, whilst the auditorium had a decorative scheme of blue and gold, and re-seated with more generous spacing between the rows reduced the capacity to 480. Behind the new arched proscenium bordering the ceiling, the stage was effectively illuminated by colour floodlighting, and the gold-coloured curtain opened to reveal the new perforated screen of "Pin-o-lite". At the rear of the hall a new sound chamber was fitted with the latest Western Electric equipment. In the enlarged projection room, the latest Kalee machines fitted with Taylor Hobson lenses guaranteed perfect pictures from the photographic point of view.

Mr. W. Hughes, the Trocadero manager was placed in control of the new cinema, with as house manager, Mr. H. Pickering, who had been connected with the Picturedrome since its opening in 1910, and recalled that the re-opening almost coincided with the 23rd anniversary of the building.

The Grand Opening as the Forum Cinema took place at 7.30pm on 20th May 1933 under the patronage of the Mayor and Mayoress of Southport, Councillor G.E. and Mrs Hardman, and the gross receipts of the performance were donated to the Mayor's social centres for the unemployed. For this night only special admission prices of 2/- and 1/- were charged, but thereafter these were to be 1/- and 7d in the evenings, and one price of 7d at bargain matinees. With the aim of booking films suitable for family audiences, the management chose as the opening film *Sleepless Nights,* from the successful London stage farce starring Stanley Lupino, supported in the all British programme by *The Tragedy of Everest,* a film of topical and educational interest dealing with the adventures of the Mount Everest Climbing Expedition. With regard to performance times these were daily, at 2.45pm, 6.30pm and 8.50pm, also one performance on Sunday at 8.15pm.

Despite the great improvements the Forum had strong competition from the start with five larger cinemas in the town centre, including the Trocadero, operated by the same company, Southport Amusements Ltd., who opened their leading cinema, the Grand, in 1938 about the same time as another large super-cinema, the Regal, was opened by ABC. The Forum therefore screened later runs of the more popular attractions and 'B' pictures, surviving until c1952, under the ownership of Grand Cinema (Southport) Ltd., when the rebuilding of the rear wall was necessary. At that time of low admissions the proprietors decided in favour of closure, the first in the Southport area, but it has not been possible to trace the date of this. Advertisements in the local press having ceased, the Forum's programmes were advertised only on the town's weekly entertainments card.

The building was demolished in August 1957 and despite a proposed redevelopment with shops and flats, the land remains a vacant site between the Carlton and the Prince of Wales hotels.

The Grand Opening of the Forum by Mayor and Mayoress of Southport is announced in the local press.
Advert: *Southport Visitor*

THE SOUTHPORT VISITER, SATURDAY, MAY 20, 1933

LORD STREET'S NEW CINEMA

Picturedrome Becomes the Forum

EXTENSIVE ALTERATIONS AND IMPROVEMENTS

Southport's Newest Cinema, **THE FORUM**

GRAND OPENING TONIGHT (SATURDAY) by the Mayor and Mayoress of Southport.
GROSS RECEIPTS IN AID OF THE MAYOR'S UNEMPLOYED SOCIAL CENTRES.
FOR COMFORT, SERVICE AND PICTURES, Second to None in Southport.
SOUND—WESTERN ELECTRIC.
GENERALLY ACKNOWLEDGED THE FINEST REPRODUCTION FOR TONE AND QUALITY.
GET THE FORUM HABIT!

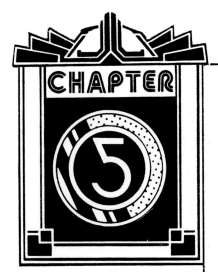

THE PICTURE PALACE/PALACE CINEMA/ESSOLDO/CLASSIC/CANNON 1 & 2
Lord Street, Southport.

Just over a year after the opening of the Picturedrome, it was announced that the Picture Palace, in a central position on Lord Street near to the Municiple Buildings was to open on 29th May 1911. Now the only surviving cinema in the Southport area, it was the first of several in the town which were designed by local architect George E. Tonge, and at that time claimed to be one of the largest purpose-built cinemas in the country with a seating capacity of 900.

The length of the building being parallel to Lord Street provided a long imposing frontage constructed of grey terra-cotta up to the verandah line and white porcelain glazed terra-cotta for the upper portion and the central tower, which was surmounted by a dome. A metal and glass verandah, 18ft. wide, extending the entire length of the building, displayed on the front, changeable white letters advertising the current attractions in addition to the cinema name, the cafe and admission prices. A feature of the verandah, which provided shelter for large numbers of people waiting to gain admission, was the absence of supporting columns. The frontage included three entrances, the central main entrance was for patrons of the stalls and boxes,those for the front stalls entered at the extreme left, and both side entrances led directly to a stairway to the cafe on the upper floor. The wide entrance hall had a marble mosaic floor and beautifully tiled dado with fibrous plaster panels and frieze above and included the pay-box and a telephone box for the use of patrons. Opposite the entrances were draped archways supported by columns beyond which entrance doors gave access to the left-hand side at the front and centre of the auditorium. Most of the seating was on one raked floor except at the rear where five boxes, each with accommodation for six people, slightly elevated above the main floor, were approached by separate staircases. The walls and ceiling were decorated with enriched fibrous plaster panels, and the entire concrete and boarded floor covered with a rich blue pile carpet.

On the upper floor, the magnificent cafe occupied the entire frontage with bay and circular windows overlooking the Boulevards and the bandstand, and it was considered that this would provide an excellent rendezvous during the summer season. Amongst the other rooms were a large boardroom, manager's and secretary's offices, ladies and gents cloakrooms, also other ante rooms, whilst the operating box of fireproof materials was constructed outside the main building, complying with the Cinematograph Act of 1909.

Kinemacolor was a process used before colour photography and cinematography, as we know it today, was developed. This photo was taken before the roof was raised and should be compared to the photo opposite where the roof line is above the central tower.
Photo: Geoff Wright

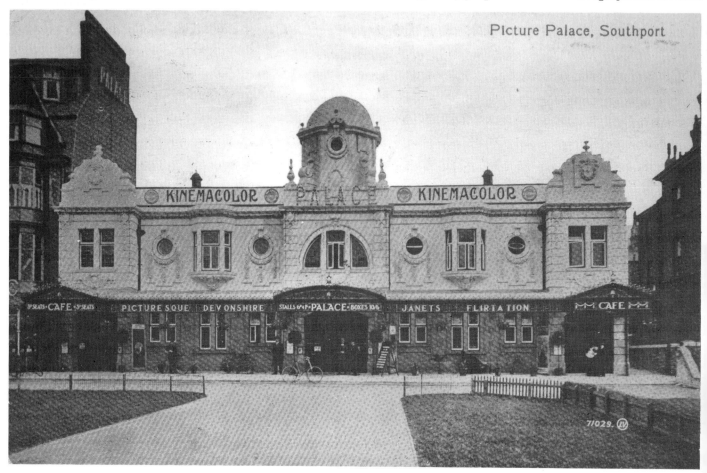

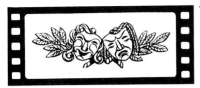

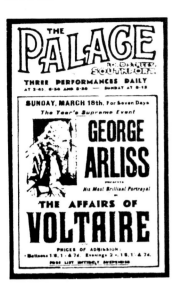

The electrical installation included two motor driven fans above the ceiling to augment the natural ventilation, and externally, 500 electric lamps were fitted to illuminate the frontage after dark.

The Picture Palace opened under the management of Mr and Mrs Charles Parker, formerly of the Empire and Pier Pavilion, who stated that every effort would be made to keep the cinema second to none in all aspects, with contracts for the most up-to-date films from the leading producers.

The Grand Opening took place on Monday 29th May 1911 with the feature film *A Tale of Two Cities* described as the finest picture of the year, also supporting short films - *Cowpuncher's Sweetheart* (Western), *Max Linder's Mother-in-Law* (Comedy), *Soap Bubbles, Baby's Fall, Rolling, Rolling,* and *Latest Motor Fiend.* Music was provided by the Bijou Orchestra which included a magnificent Broadwood grand piano, and played all the latest popular numbers.

The opening and subsequent performances were at 3pm, 7pm and 9pm, also a special matinee every Saturday morning at 11am, and one performance on Sunday at 8.15pm. Admission was at 3d, 6d and 1/- and for 10/6d, a box with six seats, all bookable in advance. Refreshments were provided free at the matinee, and there was a change of programme every Sunday, Monday and Thursday.

For many years, this was one of the town's best attended cinemas, but in 1929 when the "talkies" had commenced at three of the opposition halls, the Scala, Trocadero and Coliseum, the Palace closed for major re-construction, screening the last silent programme on 15th October - *Someone to Love* featuring Charles Rogers, also John Stuart and Brigitte Helm in *Yacht of the Seven Sins.*

Immediately the workmen moved in to begin the demolition of the interior, and in the plan of re-construction by George E. Tonge, architect of the original plans, the principal item was the raising of the entire roof bodily for the addition of a balcony, a unique and difficult operation, which was carried out by thirty-six men operating eighteen hand-jacks. Slowly, ten inches at each operation the roof was raised 17ft. 6ins. above the former level, a feat which attracted large crowds from all over the north-west, who watched the operation with amazement.

The provision of an increase in the seating capacity to 1,053 was the chief reason that the alterations were decided upon, as the seating accommodation was not sufficient to warrant the enormous expense of the new Western Electric Talking equipment. At the request of Western Electric many innovations were made to improve the acoustics of the auditorium into which a specially designed control room opened, and deeply coffered panels were fixed to the entire ceiling, which not only improved the acoustics, but also gave a distinguished and impressive note to the interior.

The present Cannon cinema is one of Merseyside's oldest operating cinemas. The frontage, even at night, was designed to attract attention and was originally illuminated after dark by 500 filament lamps. The night view was taken in 1935 after neon had replaced the filament lamps, and the daytime one in the 1950's.
Photos: Mike Taylor (right) and L. Houghton (below)

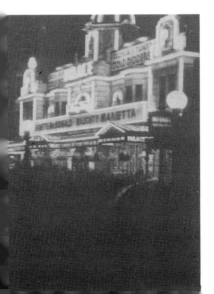

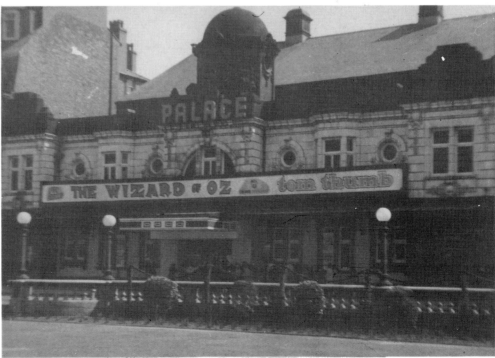

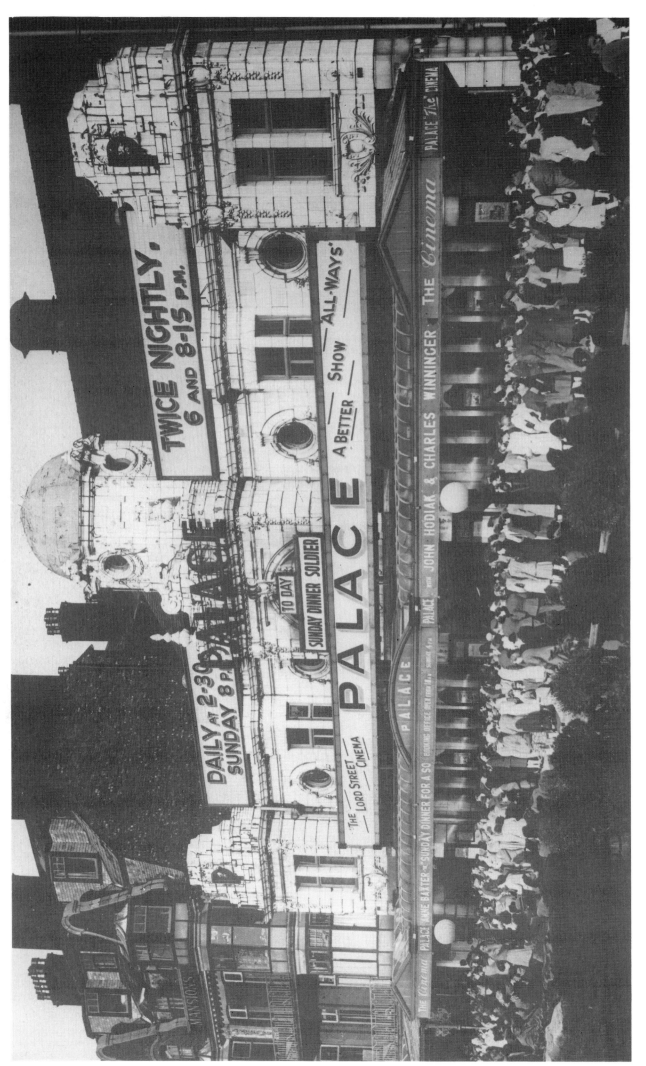

PALACE

THE LORD STREET CINEMA

DAILY AT 2·30 SUNDAY 8 P.M.

TWICE NIGHTLY, 6 AND 8·15 P.M.

A BETTER SHOW ALL·WAYS'

TO DAY SUNDAY DINNER SOLDIER

PALACE

PALACE with ANNE BAXTER · JOHN HODIAK & CHARLES WINNINGER · THE Cinema

Palace Ice Cinema

The popularity of the Palace may be gauged by this 1947 view of patrons queuing up to see *Sunday Dinner for a Soldier*.
Photo: L. Houghton

The attractive profile of the cinema is brought into sharp focus with floodlights in this night view below.

32

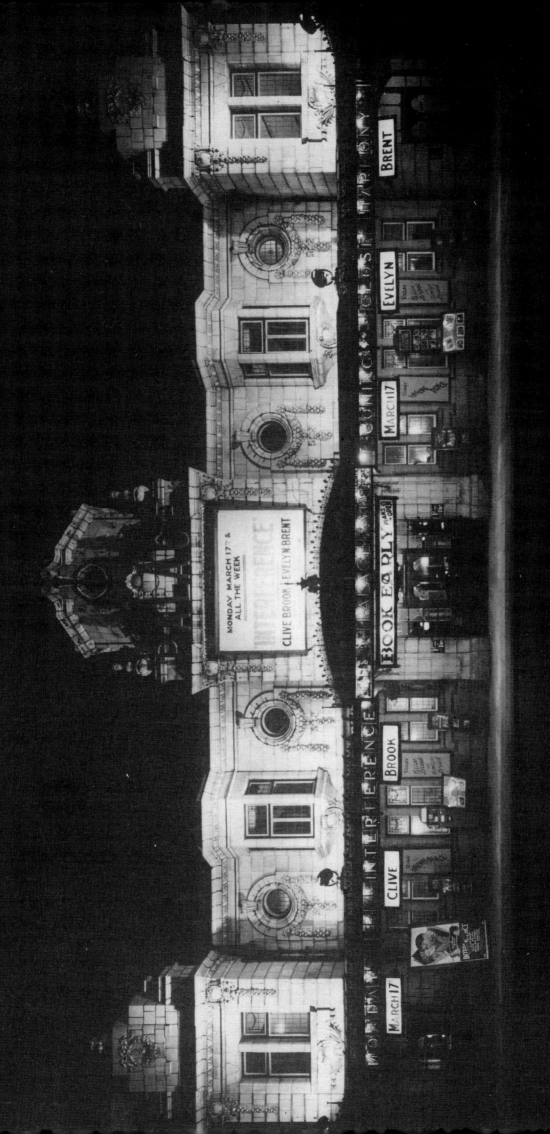

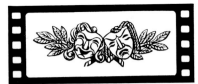

The circle lounge which replaced the first-floor cafe.
Photo: L. Houghton

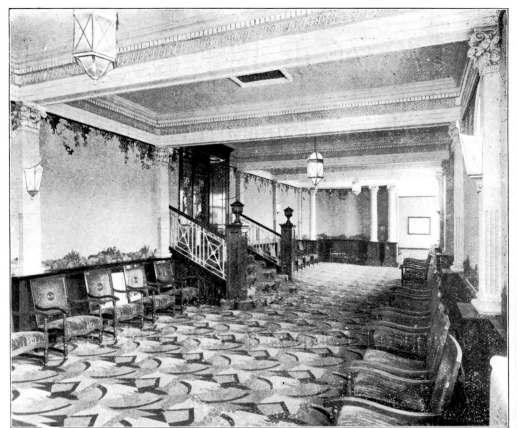

The beautiful decorations were predominantly of old ivory and gold, and a special feature was the elegance of the proscenium opening, surmounted by a painting of sea horses in classical design which occupied the whole of the space above, with the exception of the centre, where the Southport coat-of-arms was in an honoured position. The draperies of the proscenium and doors were in a rich heavy velvet relieved with a wide braid in contrasting colours of blue and flame.

The principal illumination was by a huge central lantern suspended from the high, curved ceiling, with glass sections lit from within, whilst around the edge were torch-shaped light fittings. Subsidiary lighting was in the form of demi-coups on the pilasters of the walls and deck lights beneath the circle ceiling, which also incorporated a wide dome with suspended glass shaded light fitting and ventilation shaft above. In this rear part of the stalls, the former boxes were replaced by seats on a stepped floor extending up to the rear wall, there being no crossover gangway, entrances and exits being along the side walls.

Replacing the cafe on the first floor, the luxurious lounge was described as one of the charms of the alterations with rows of comfortable armchairs, and a luxurious carpet.Entered as before by a stairway at either end, this now included the entrances to the new circle, and the principal one of these was in the centre where the doors were at the head of a short flight of stairs with gold-painted balustrade, and at the foot, lanterns mounted on square columns. The doors gave access to the left-hand side of the circle which had side promenades, each with fourteen single seats,leading to the exits at the front of the hall. This enabled patrons to leave the building without having to pass through the waiting room, which could accommodate a capacity circle audience.

Advertised as the most handsome and most comfortable cinema in the North, the Grand Re-opening as the Palace was by The Mayor of Southport, Alderman A. Tomlinson, J. P. at 8pm on Monday, 3 March 1930, when the feature film, a star attraction of that year and Paramount's first musical, was the All talking, Singing and Dancing *Innocents of Paris* featuring Maurice Chevalier. Subsequent performances were at 2.45pm, 6.40pm, and 8.50pm to which admission was at 2/-, 1/6d, 1/- and 6d, and in view of the anticipated heavy rush for tickets patrons were advised to book their seats in advance at the box office open from 10am to 10pm.

Having seen the growth and decline of silent films, the Palace then entered the second phase of its long career with the miracle of the "Talkies" and under the control of the local independent company Associated Southport Cinemas Ltd. continued to provide for thousands of film fans despite the opening by Gaumont British of a large super cinema,

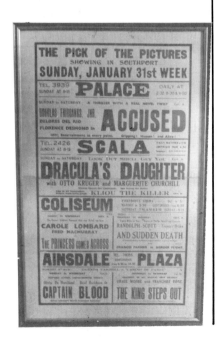

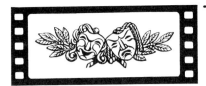

The new auditorium looking from
the screen to the circle.
Photo: L. Houghton

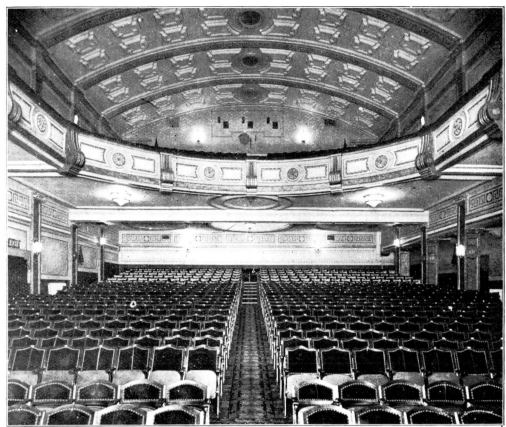

the Palladium, only 8 months later, followed 8 years later by the opening of the Grand, and the Regal, an ABC cinema.

Notable presentations during the thirties were screened at a series of midnight matinees including a gala performance of *The King Steps Out* starring the opera singer Grace Moore.

In the late forties the Palace specialised in long-running films when it was unusual to retain a film for a second week, and in this period *The Best Years of our Lives* ran for eight weeks, and a Danny Kaye film for five. The cinema also saw the world premiere of Carol Reed's screen classic *The Third Man* and the first public showing in Britain of *Jazz on a Summer's Day* which attracted audiences from miles away.

But the Palace's greatest hour was probably in being chosen as the first independent cinema in the country to play the late Mike Todd's *Around the World in Eighty Days*. Plans of the building had to be sent to America for approval and a special screen, lenses and minor mechanical parts installed for the occasion, This was justified by the fact that the film ran in 1958 for 11 weeks, and was brought back for another two weeks later in the year, a record run for Southport but it transpired that even this was to be beaten. After closing on 25 June 1966 with the programme - *Ride beyond Vengeance* and *That Man in Istanbul* there was partial modernisation and the installation of the town's first 70mm equipment and multi-track stereophonic sound, opening on 4 July 1966 with *My Fair Lady* starring Rex Harrison and Audrey Hepburn, which beat the previous record, playing for sixteen weeks. There were separate performances and advance booking with admission prices at 12/6d in the circle, and 10/6d and 7/6d in the stalls.

For about 12 months from March 1971 under the control of the Newcastle-based Essoldo cinema circuit the Palace was re-named the Essoldo, then taken over by Classic Cinemas Ltd. who restored the name Palace during its last two years as a single screen cinema.

Early in 1974 work began on an £80,000 modernisation scheme providing two cinemas, the stalls with 500 seats formed Classic 1 with, at the rear, a newly constructed projection room equipped with a Westrex projector and sound, also a "Tower" long running system. Above, the balcony, extended to the front with an additional 200 seats became Classic 2 with 400 seats. This was served by the original projection room with Fedi 35/70mm projectors and RCA stereo sound. The work, which included new carpets, complete re-decoration and refurbishment was surprisingly completed without loss of performances, which remained continuous daily.

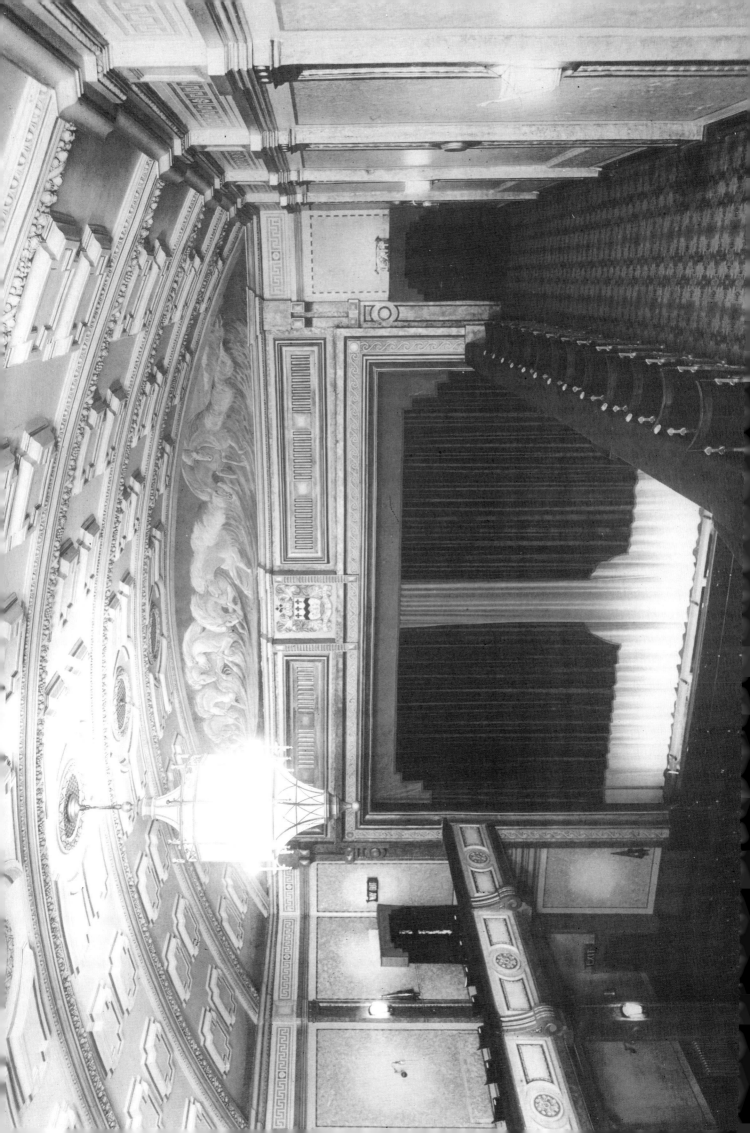

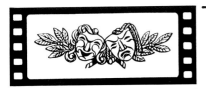

Opposite: The imposing square-shaped proscenium, surmounted by the Southport coat-of-arms and the painting of seahorses, the width of the auditorium.
Photo: John Maltby

The twin Cinemas opened as Classic 1 & 2 on 12 May 1974, when screening in Classic 1. *A Touch of Class* featured Glenda Jackson and George Segal, supported by *If It's Tuesday, This Must Be Belgium* whilst in Classic 2. Bruce Lee starred in *The Big Boss* supported by *The Love Machine*.

External modernisation consisted of frameless glass doors in the main entrance, and a new canopy surmounted by an internally-illuminated lettering display sign, divided in the centre to advertise the films in No. 1 and No.2 cinemas. At this time the frontage was minus the central tower removed in 1972 as unsafe.

Towards the end of 1988 the twin cinemas were improved by a £280,000 renovation including a re-styled foyer, new carpets, seating and central heating together with extensive re-decoration.

Now with its 80th anniversary in the not too distant future, the cinema is among the longest surviving in the country, and the recent major improvements indicate the confidence of the proprietors in a long future ahead for Cannon 1 & 2, the only remaining commercial cinemas in the area between the Liverpool suburbs and Preston.

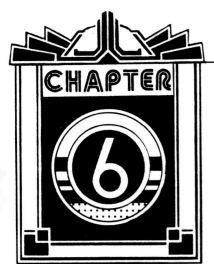

CHAPTER 6

TIVOLI PICTURE PALACE/QUEEN'S CINEMA, Devonshire Road, High Park

Prior to conversion into a cinema in 1912, the building was used by the Liberal Party as a Club. The 31 ft. wide frontage resembled a double-fronted dwelling house with a double door in the centre within an arched entranceway, whilst on either side was a splay bay window. The frontage of red brick had at first-floor level, three tall windows in the centre and the upper part formed a steep gable.

Internally there was a central entrance hall 6ft. wide and numerous rooms constituting living accommodation, above which a meeting hall occupied the floor above. In 1912 plans were drawn up by Ernest W. Ball & Son, Chartered Surveyors of Southport for the conversion of the upper floor into a small cinema. At the far end of the entrance hall a pay-box was constructed and immediately on the right of this, the former stairway with a right-hand turn led up to the entrance at the front of the auditorium on the left-hand side. The enclosed stairway and gangways around it resulted in some loss of seating in this part of the hall where the first seven rows of seats were shorter. The auditorium, 51ft by 31ft, had a seating capacity of 305 with a gangway along either side, and a central gangway divided the longer rows into two blocks of seats. At the rear, an exit door at either side led to a stairway to ground level, to which there was also access from the sides of the newly constructed projection room, an extension of the first floor supported by cantilevers.

Under the same ownership as the Picturedrome, Lord Street, the cinema opened as the Tivoli Picture Palace on 20th May 1912, when the local press reported that the old Liberal Club had been transformed into a cosy and comfortable Palace of Delight! The hall was crowded with an enthusiastic audience for the opening performance at 7.45pm to see the programme of films entitled - *The Baby Show* (comedy), *The General's Daughter* (war drama), *Hilda's Lovers*, *The Innkeeper's Daughter*, *Yellowstone Joe* and *Cat and Dog* (cartoon). Admission prices at 3d, 4d and 6d, reduced to 2d and 3d for children were probably the lowest in the Southport area. Performances were to be at 7.45pm every evening except Saturday and Sunday, the former with three performances at 2.30pm, 6.30pm and 8.45pm, whilst on Sunday there was a performance at 8.15pm.

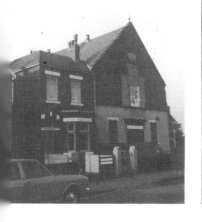

The Queen's, High Park, in use as a club.
Photo: Tony Moss

The cinema name was changed to the Queen's c1920 under the ownership of High Park Picture Palace Co. (Southport) Ltd., who appointed as resident manager, Mr Alexander Knight, who in 1925 took over the lease of the Picturedrome, Formby.

Five years later, in 1930, the cinema was considerably altered and improved, again to the plans of Ernest W. Ball and Son, which on the ground floor eliminated the front rooms on either side of the hall to create an entrance hall the full width of the building, from which the cinema was entered by a stairway at either side from the main entrance doors. After turning and ascending adjacent to the sides of the building, a double door at the head gave access near the front of the auditorium at either side, where between the enclosed stairways were fitted several shorter rows of seats. With side gangways only, the seating capacity was then reduced to 251, but this was due to several shorter rows also at the rear to provide wider gangways.

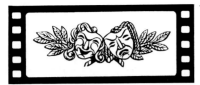

The top elevation shows the building when used as a club by the Liberal Party. The one below is when it was converted into the Tivoli, High Park. Elevations: Ashby Ball

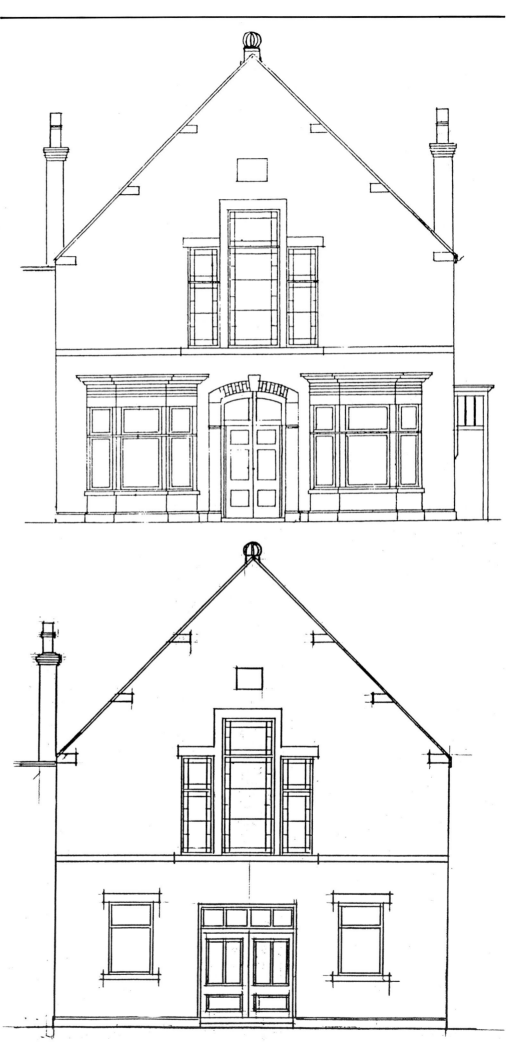

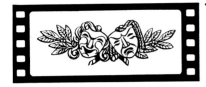

The projection area was also improved by a door at the rear leading on to a stairway to a film rewinding room below, whereas previously the inflammable nitrate film had to be taken outside the box to a room on the ground floor. This is said to have caused the problem of rainwater occasionally damaging the films, resulting in complaints from the suppliers.

Under the same ownership during the late forties, the seating capacity was only 213, accounted for by the bringing forward of the screen to provide space for the speaker at the rear when AWH sound system was installed c1931.

In its later years of the forties and fifties, the Queen's was open for two performances in the evening with admission at 6d to 1/6d and there were four changes of programme weekly, as a remaining small independent cinema restricted to older films.

At closure in 1957 the building was converted for use as the High Park Labour Club, after which during the seventies a local resident acquired it, and reverting to the original name, the Tivoli, ran it as a private members' club, until near the end of the decade when the present use was commenced as the Southport Post Office and Telecommunications social club. This includes a licensed bar on the ground floor, and above, the former cinema has a small dance floor with tables, chairs around, and a licensed bar.

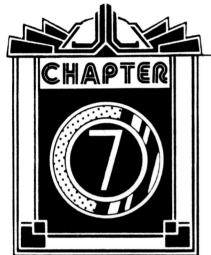

PICTUREDROME/QUEEN'S CINEMA, Three Tuns Lane, Formby

The building was originally constructed as a Club house by the Catholic Association, which was registered as a limited company on 15th August 1893. It was planned by the school architects, erected at a cost of £498 and opened by Monseignor Carr on 13th October 1894. During subsequent years, additions and alterations to the building were made and, in 1912, Monseignor Carr, who was concerned that there was little in the district to occupy young people in the evening, pressed for its conversion into a cinema. Plans for the conversion of the building, then the Formby Catholic Club, were drawn up and in October 1912, Monseignor Carr made the first of several applications to the Formby court for a cinematograph and music licence. At least the first two were unsuccessful since the plans did not completely satisfy the conditions of the Cinematograph Act of 1909, and although there is no record of the date when the licence was granted, the cinema was operational in December 1912 by which time Monseignor Carr had resigned his position due to ill health.

The local press of 21st December 1912 announced the cinema was NOW OPEN with Special Holiday Programme, twice nightly at 6.45pm and 8.45pm, also a matinee on Wednesday at 3.00pm and a children's matinee on Saturday at 2.30pm. The films were entitled *The Emperor's Message* (a stirring Napoleonic drama), *The Gun Smugglers, Game Shooting from Aeroplane* and *The Drummer Girl from Vicksburg* (a stirring war drama), also Journal of Current Events etc. The admission prices of 3d, 6d and 1/- were in accordance with those at the majority of cinemas at that time.

Electricity was brought to Formby with the opening of the Picturedrome, the generator at the rear also supplying current to several houses nearby, but with the disadvantage that the house lights went out when the cinema closed!

The Picturedrome had a small stadium-style auditorium, approximately 60ft by 25ft with seating for nearly 200 patrons, whilst on the first floor was the club room, completely cut off from the cinema in accordance with licensing regulations, with separate entrance and exits.

The cinema continued in its original form until 1925 by which time the upper floor had been converted into a dance hall under the ownership of Union, Bradford and Fenton. In 1925 the building was leased to Mr. Alexander Knight, who, considering that Formby should possess a theatre in keeping with its growing importance as a residential centre, engaged Southport architect Mr. Ernest W. Ball, FSI, AMICE to design and supervise a major scheme of reconstruction and alterations. The principal object of this was to considerably increase the seating capacity by dispensing with the dance hall and utilising the space for the construction of a balcony with 115 seats reached by a stairway from a separate entrance on the frontage, whilst at the rear of the balcony a new and enlarged operating box was provided. Near the front on the left-hand side an exit led to a newly constructed stairway to ground level outside the main building.

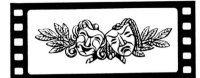

Externally, the comfort of patrons was considered by the erection of a verandah above the separate stalls and balcony entrances at either side of the pay-box. On the right-hand side, two pairs of doors in the vestibule gave access to the rear stalls crossover gangway, and on this floor were 198 seats with a gangway along either side.

Alexander Knight announced the Grand re-opening of the cinema, re-named the Queen's on Tuesday, 29th December 1925 at 7.30pm with an exceptional programme including a Star Picture, supporting film programme and artistes, Mr. R. Nutter, Baritone, Mr. Bert Stanbury, Humorist and Entertainer also the Popular Professional Orchestra.

Mr. Knight ran the cinema for just three years until December 1928, when he was killed when his car was set on fire while transporting inflammable nitrate film.

The change over to the "talkies" came rather late to the Queen's, which advertised in the latter half of 1930 - "When all is said and done, Silence is Golden - Come to the Queen's". In October of that year, Kalee 7 projectors and B.T.P. sound system were installed for the opening on Monday 13th of the Vitaphone Talking Picture *Smiling Irish Eyes* featuring Colleen Moore, also supporting programme including the *Universal Talking News* with commentary by the famous R.E. Jeffrey. Featured in a complete change of programme for the latter half of the week, *Atlantic* with Franklyn Dyall was the story of the liner *Titanic*.

During the 1930's the cinema was leased to Philip M. Hanmer of the Liverpool-based Regent Enterprise circuit who ran it until final closure in 1957. First closing in 1953, then re-opening for a short time 1957/58, the Queen's having a proscenium width of only 14ft was completely unsuitable for the wide screen systems of the 1950's and restricted the choice of films which could be shown.

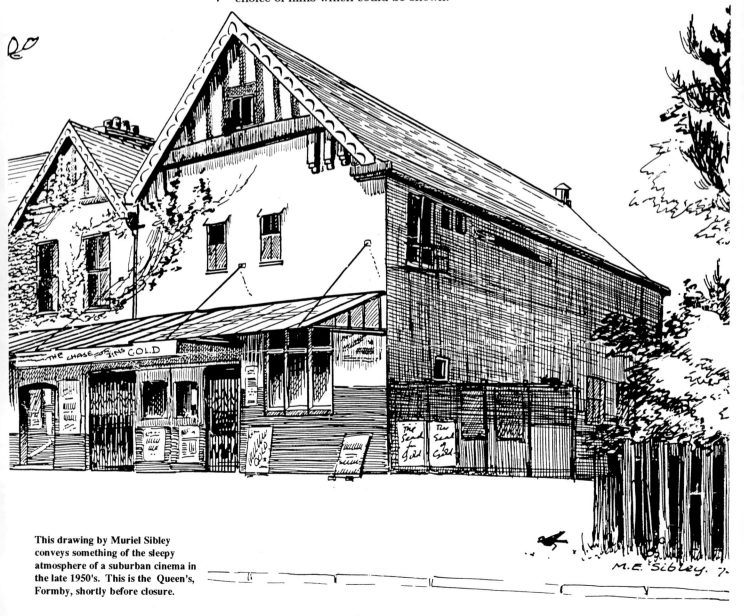

This drawing by Muriel Sibley conveys something of the sleepy atmosphere of a suburban cinema in the late 1950's. This is the Queen's, Formby, shortly before closure.

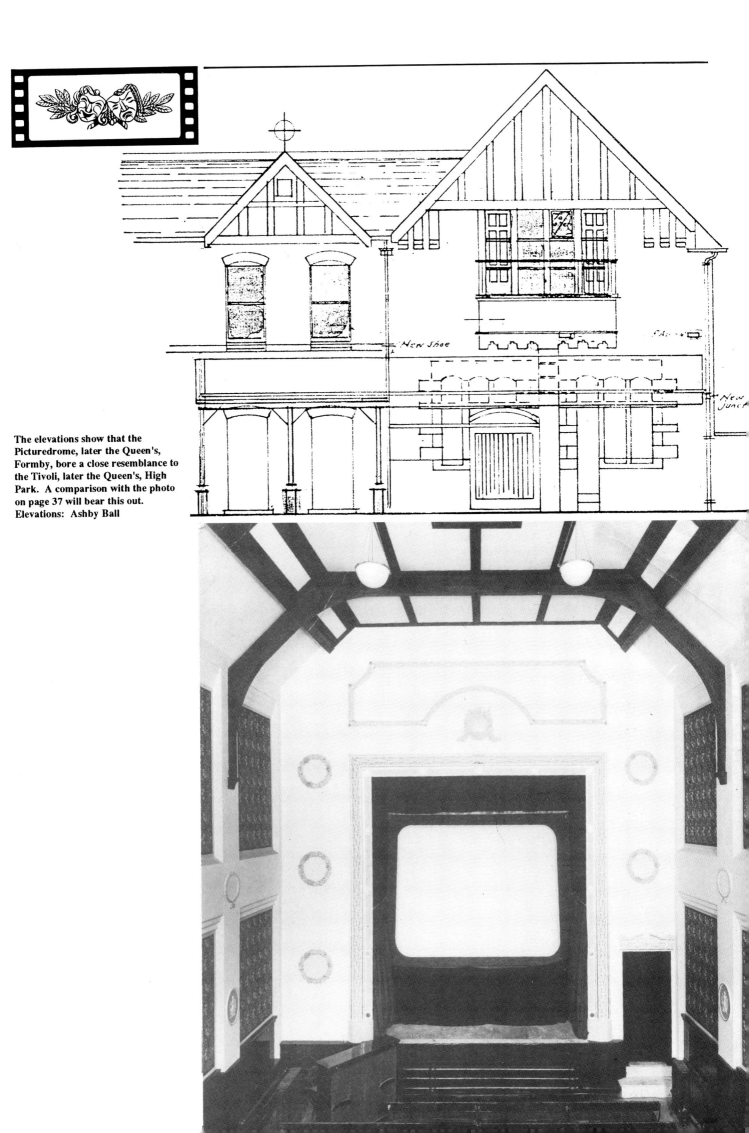

The elevations show that the Picturedrome, later the Queen's, Formby, bore a close resemblance to the Tivoli, later the Queen's, High Park. A comparison with the photo on page 37 will bear this out.
Elevations: Ashby Ball

New Shoe

New Junc

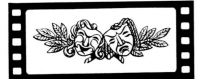

A 1925 announcement in the *Southport Visitor* tells the public that the Picturedrome is now the Queen's. Below is the inevitable end of so many suburban cinemas. Photo: Mrs. Yorke, The Formby Society

MR. ALEXANDER KNIGHT

Begs to announce

GRAND RE-OPENING

OF THE

QUEEN'S CINEMA, FORMBY,

On TUESDAY NEXT, December 29th, at 7-30 p.m.

The Exceptional Programme will include

A STAR PICTURE, Etc.

ARTISTES:

Mr. R. NUTTER, Baritone;   The Popular Professional Orchestra;

Mr. BERT STANBURY, Humorist and Entertainer.

After final closure as a cinema in 1958, the hall was used for short periods as a skating rink and a jazz club, after which it stood empty for a considerable time until demolition in the sixties when the building and site were acquired by the Co-operative Society who opened the new building as a supermarket. This later came under the ownership of Fine Fare and after a period of closure it was Hanbury's supermarket. The present owners Ethel Austin & Co. Ltd took over in 1987, adding it to their chain of stores.

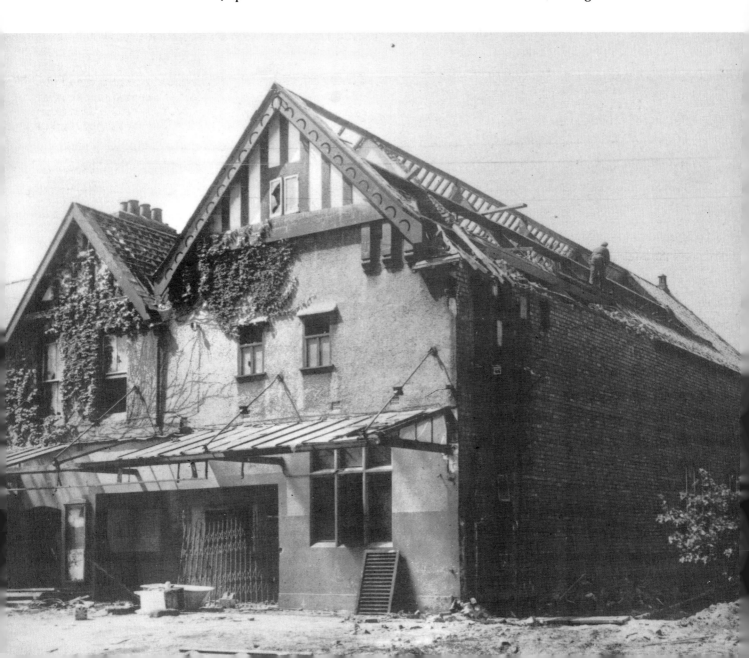

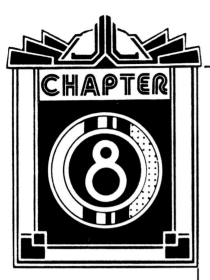

CHAPTER 8

THE PICTURE HOUSE/COLISEUM CINEMA, Nevill Street, Southport

The town's third purpose-built cinema was erected upon what was described as practically an 'island' site on Nevill Street, which linked Lord Street with the promenade. To the plans of Gilbert Wilson, a Southport architect, it was a stadium-type auditorium with accommodation for 750 people.

The mainly plaster-covered facade was relieved above the full width glass verandah, by vertical sections of stonework extending up to the coping at either side and flanking the windows of the first floor. These consisted of, in the centre, the two half circular windows of the cafe, whilst at either side, a small circular window was set within a stonework surround. The highest part of the frontage was adorned at either side by a stone balustrade. In the centre, two arched entrance ways, with two pairs of glass-panelled doors at the head of the steps gave access to the foyer with walls decorated by white plaster above a 4ft dado of mahogany. From this, doors at either side led into the rear of the auditorium in which most of the seating was on a raked floor with the exception of four boxes on a raised floor at the rear, a scheme similar to that which had been carried out at the Picture Palace, Lord Street.

The auditorium ceiling was stated to be considerably higher than at the majority of picture theatres, and following its contours, the arched proscenium made possible a larger than average picture, which measured 19ft by 17ft at a distance from the projection room of 102 ft, then the longest picture 'throw' in Southport. Two projectors of the latest type were installed in the operating box, constructed of fireproof brazed concrete slabs, three inches thick, had an armoured fireproof door. But should fire break out, steel shutters would automatically drop over the projection ports, through which the pictures were shown.

Illumination of the auditorium was by the new semi-indirect method of bowl-shaped shades, which directed the light from the electric globes upwards to the ceiling, and at the end of performances, sudden glare was avoided, the lights being gradually turned on by dimmers. The heating arrangements were installed under the supervision of the Southport Corporation gas engineer and it was stated that in connection with the perfect, modern ventilating system, the architect had arranged for an air duct to run up from underneath the floor in the centre gangway through gratings for warm air in various positions, and for the removal of foul air, an unusually large central heating fan, 36 inches in diameter was fitted above the auditorium ceiling.

The Picture House was opened to the public without formal ceremony on Saturday 13th May 1913, when the continuous performance was from 10.45am to 10.30pm. The feature film *Zaza* (coloured) was supported by a programme of short films including *The Black League* and *Ceylon* (coloured) stated to be the latest and finest films available. It was reported that large numbers of people attended throughout the day and were full of praise for the programme and the comfort of the auditorium. In line with the town's other cinemas, admission prices were 3d, 6d and 1/- with half prices for children in the 6d and 1/- seats until 5pm. The cafe was in the course of construction and opened a few weeks later.

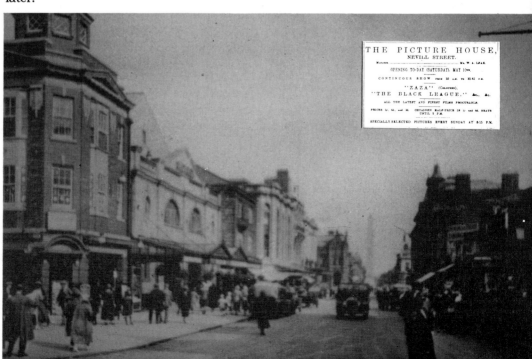

The Picture House, later the Coliseum.
Photo: Tony Moss

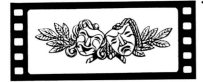

Before the end of 1913, the Picture House had the distinction of presenting for the first time in Southport the very latest improvement in the cinema world - "Talking Pictures by the Edison Kinetophone", one of only eight such installations throughout the country, Southport then being regarded in cinema circles as a first class town. Just before Christmas 1913, press representatives were invited for a private viewing of the system, with which the sound from a gramophone record was synchronised with the speech or action of the film, although not with constant accuracy! It was reported that the principal film *Her Redemption* would have been poor without the Kinetophone, and there were supporting films in the programme entitled *After College Days* (comedy) and *The Soldiers' Chorus* from Faust.

The fame of the Edison Kinetophone soon spread and there were crowded houses for the opening to the public on Monday, 22nd December 1913 with performances at 3pm, 5pm, 7pm and 9pm for which patrons were advised to book their seats in advance. The two talking pictures were *The Edison Lectures* and *The Edison Minstrels*. The former told of the advantages of the novelty, by which the voices of great singers, actors and orators would be heard in the years to come, whilst during the latter, the singing, joking and laughter of the performers were heard.

Silent films constituted the remainder of the programme, comprising of *Babes in the Wood* an adaptation of the fairy tale, two dramas, *Red Falcon* and *The Compact*, a comedy, *Slippery Pimple*, a colour travel film and *Pathe Gazette* of topical events. Admission prices remained as at the opening.

Edison's talking pictures proved to be a great novelty attraction and the season of these lasted until the end of March 1914, after which silent films were shown until closing on 21st January 1922 with *The Mystery of Bernard Brown* by Phillips Oppenheim.

The hall was closed for almost one month for extensive alterations, additions and re-decoration on an elaborate scale, which it was stated reflected the enterprising policy of Mr. William Walker, the manager and secretary for many years since transferring from

Three char-a-bancs are lined up outside the Coliseum, as the Picture House was re-named in 1922.
Photo: Metropolitan Borough of Sefton (D. Taylor, Attractions Department)

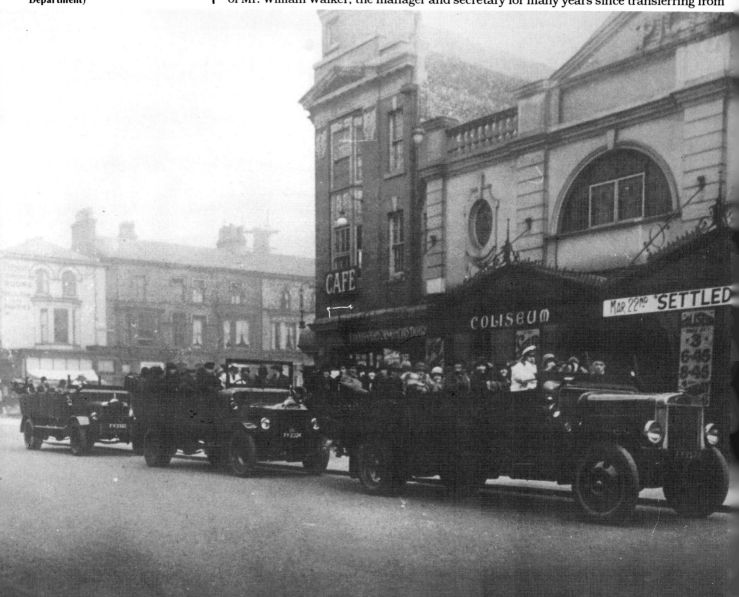

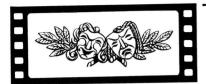

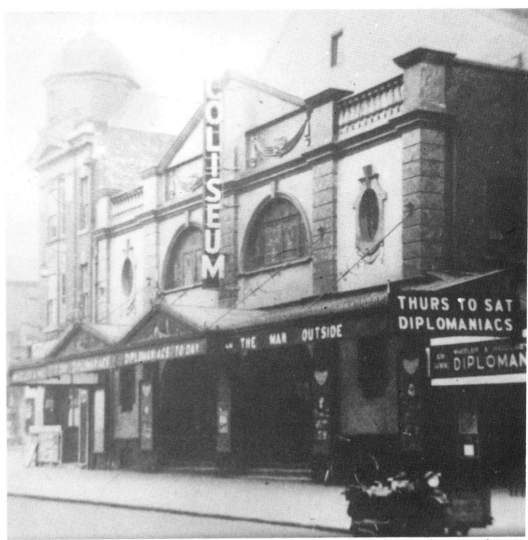

The ornate frontage of the Coliseum, typical of those built before World War I.
Photo: W.E. Marsden

the position of general manager at the zoo and skating rink in the Winter Gardens complex. In the re-styled auditorium a seating capacity of 1,000 was achieved by the addition of several rows of seats, which replaced the boxes at the rear, and seven exits enabled the hall, when full, to be cleared within three minutes in case of emergency.

Originally owned by a company known as the Nevill Street Picture House (Southport) Ltd, there was at this time a change of proprietor to the Coliseum Cinema (Southport) Ltd, and re-opening on Saturday 18th February 1922 was as the Coliseum the Cinema Superba. A special programme for the day was headed by the Famous-Lasky film *The Great Day* with a star cast headed by Arthur Bouchier, the Shakespearian actor. A company of musicians formed the Grand Harmonic Orchestra under the direction of Mr. Edward Beck direct from the Scala, Liverpool. The three performances were at 2.00pm, 6.45pm and 8.45pm , Sunday at 8.15pm. Prices of admission were then - Grand Stalls 1/3d, Stalls 1/- (bookable in advance) and Front seats 6d.

Available information suggests that the Picture House had an organ from about 1921, one of only two in Southport cinemas, the other being at the Palladium, Lord Street. Announcing the re-opening as the Coliseum, it was stated that Mr. R.K.D. Bannister would be retained as the organist. The two-manual console of light oak, situated in the orchestra pit in front of the stage, was described as a fine instrument, with two keyboards identical in arrangement to that of a church organ, which was to be its eventual use after being sold to a church in Yorkshire in 1932. Organ interludes ceased in 1931, when for about five years the organist had been J. Wilfred Clayton. By this time the "talkies" were well established at the Coliseum, Western Electric sound system having been installed for the opening on 7th October 1929 of the first all-talking British film *Blackmail* directed by Alfred Hitchcock and starring John Longden and Anny Ondra. Intending patrons were advised to book their seats early and admission prices were then 6d to 2/6d.

The Coliseum continued under the management of Mr. William Walker until 1930, and during his regime he had been successful in securing the cream of the world's pictures, also booking for the Palace, Southport and the Plaza, Ainsdale. Notable films included *Intolerance*, *Way Down East* and *The Four Horsemen of the Apocalypse*.

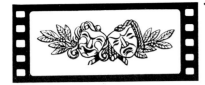

The cinemas of Coliseum (Southport) Ltd. came under the control of the newly formed company Associated Southport Cinemas, c1935, when an extensive exterior and interior modernisation of the Coliseum was commenced. The frontage was re-styled on the plain modern lines of the thirties with a facing of glazed faience tiles, in buff colour up to the canopy level and cream above. The upper part was relieved by a tall central fin bearing on either side, vertically, the name COLISEUM illuminated by neon tubes, and there were also several tall narrow windows. The old glass verandah was replaced by a plain black painted canopy above the four separate entrance ways, each with a double glass panelled door with metal adornments. At either side of the entrances, two very large, upright still frames were fitted flush with the tiles.

The auditorium and foyer also received a 1930's treatment with plain, light coloured surfaces, and in the foyer, a modern pay-box was fitted flush with the wall opposite the entrance doors. In the auditorium, at either side of the proscenium, a splayed wall with ventilation grille was constructed above the front stalls exits, and for the greater comfort of patrons, re-seating reduced the capacity to 835.

In 1938 two new super cinemas, the Grand and the Regal had been added to the already formidable competition in the town, resulting in the Coliseum being restricted to a selection of older films and "B" pictures including a regular series of cowboy films, for which often most of the seats were filled by local teenagers and so many of these films were shown that the cinema was nicknamed the "Ranch House".

In the mid-1930's a streamlined facade was grafted on to the frontage and internally the auditorium and foyer were given a modern finish.
Photo: Norman Green

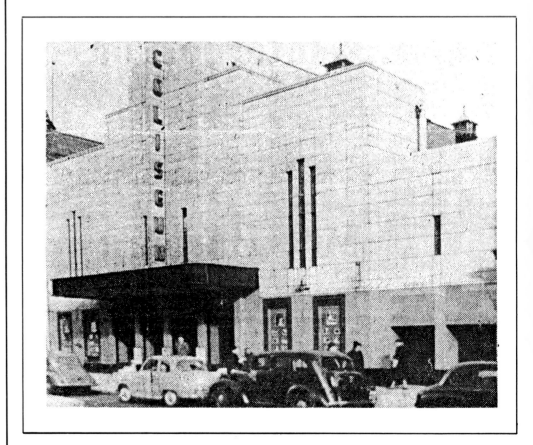

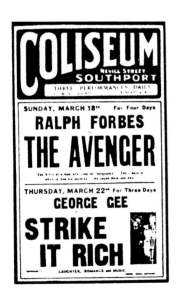

The decline in attendances during the fifties was continuing when in 1957 there was a final change of ownership to the Emery Cinema circuit of Blackpool, whose managing director, Mr. Gordon Emery, in an attempt to attract new audiences, announced a new policy of screening the best Continental films. This was not successful and on 21st October 1959, the local press announced the closure of the Coliseum on 14th November. The reason given by Mr. Emery was that Southport was overcrowded with entertainments in the winter, although the chief competition was from television. The final programme at the Coliseum was a double feature - *Tabarin* featuring Sylvia Lopez and *Backlash* with Richard Widmark.

The site was sold to a London group for re-development as shops, but for many years the major portion has been occupied by an amusement arcade.

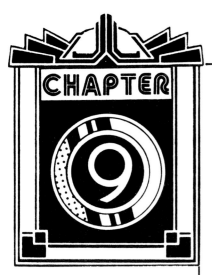

THE BIRKDALE PICTURE PALACE, Upper Aughton Road, Birkdale

This small purpose-built cinema near to the junction of Upper Aughton Road and Mosely Street opened on the same day, 13th May 1913 as the Picture House, Nevill Street. The building was stated to be fireproof and up-to-date in every respect, and an outstanding feature was the method of construction, the roof being supported by steel stanchions with the result that the brick walls were only a filling to the structure. The length of this was parallel to the road, but angled back towards the left-hand side providing space for the entrance and a small foyer between the frontage and the auditorium. This was stated to have the advantage of giving direct access to the better seats at the rear, which would not have been possible had the entrance been centralised. The quite long single storey frontage was faced with white cement and included several tall windows of the various ground floor areas. Flanked by fluted pilasters, the entrance was in the form of a high archway in which the upper part was of small three-cornered sections of glass. The two entrance doors each had a large panel of glass forming a pattern, and brass handles, whilst above was a sign bearing the word ENTRANCE in large white letters, also the proprietors name - The Birkdale Picture Palace Limited.

THE BIRKDALE PICTURE PALACE,
UPPER AUGHTON ROAD
(CORNER WALTON ROAD)
MANAGER .... MR. A WADE
GRAND OPENING TO - DAY
(SATURDAY), AT 3 O'CLOCK.
JAMES PATTERSON. DETECTIVE, &c., &c
THREE PERFORMANCES—
3, 7, AND 9 DAILY, DURING WHIT-WEEK.
PICTURES CHANGED TWICE WEEKLY
SUNDAYS 8.15—SPECIAL PROGRAMME
PRICES OF ADMISSION—Stalls, 3d.; 2nd Seats, 4d.; 7d. 3d. MATINEES—3d, 4d, 2d.

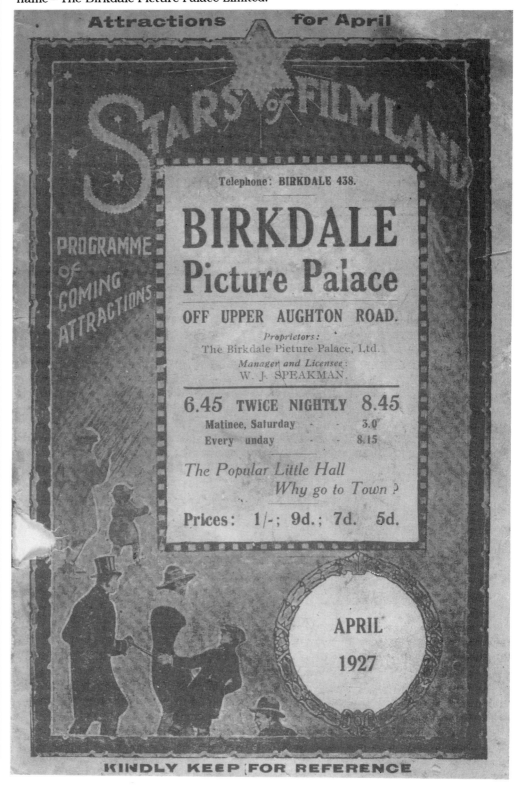

The Birkdale Picture Palace opened the same day as the Coliseum, 13th May 1913. Although only a small cinema it provided an attractive programme of forthcoming attractions.
Programme: Chris Robey

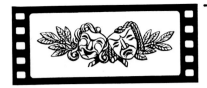

Beyond the entrance doors the foyer had a 4ft dado of mahogany, whilst the remainder of the treatment was in white plaster, and the decorations throughout were described as pleasing, subdued colours having been introduced.

From the foyer, direct access was to the right-hand side at the rear of the stadium-type auditorium with a seating capacity of 450, of which the better seats at the rear were tip-up chairs, the cheaper seats at the front consisted of forms, reached by a separate entrance, and the floor was covered by a handsome Axminster carpet. Four exits were provided and considered ample since the building could be cleared in 60 seconds.

It was noted that the contour of the ceiling was greater than in the majority of cinemas, and following this the proscenium arch enabled a larger picture size of 14ft by 12ft by two of the latest Pathe projectors installed in the separately-constructed operating box in accordance with the 1909 Cinematograph Act.

A feature of the auditorium was that no encroachment of the side gangways had been made by pilasters, the ornamental ceiling ribs tied on the cornices, the latter being supported by ornamental consoles. Between these, the decoration was by plaster panels and it was stated that the whole treatment had produced effective results.

Reporting the opening, the local press stated that the building had been completed in a manner which should give the greatest satisfaction not only to the management but to patrons who would no doubt fill the house nightly.

The Grand Opening under the management of Mr. A. Wade was at 3.00pm on Saturday, 10th May 1913 with the feature film *James Patterson, Detective*, also supporting shorts entitled - *Woodland, A Bit of Blue Ribbon, On the Steps of the Throne* and *Making A Hero of Her*. Evening performances were at 7.00pm and 9.00pm, which were to be the normal times except Sunday with one performance at 8.15pm, and matinees were restricted to Tuesday and Saturday only at 3.00pm. Lower than admission prices in the town, the rear stalls were 9d, second stalls 6d and pit 3d, which were reduced to 6d, 4d and 2d at the matinees. Patrons received a free programme for *The World Before Your Eyes Entertainment* of which there was a complete change of programme every Sunday, Monday and Thursday, and were advised that the proprietors had spared no expense in the beautiful decorations and upholstery, which made it one of the cosiest and most up-to-date Picture Theatres in Lancashire.

Musical accompaniment to the silent pictures was by a pianist, who picked music to suit the mood of the films, playing in the evening from 6.30pm and practising at afternoon rehearsal runs, but often when the "westerns" were shown, the children, by whom the place was called "Flick Hall", made so much noise that the piano could not be heard, so the pianist just sat back and watched the film! Popular stars of the silent screen at the Palace were Tom Mix and William S. Hart in "westerns", the dramas of Warner Oland and Ruth Roland, whilst there were roars of laughter at the comedies of Charlie Chaplin, Harold Lloyd and Buster Keaton, and Pearl White was a great favourite of the exciting serials.

The Birkdale Picture Palace was, and still is for that matter, an attractive building. The elevations, right and far right, show how finely detailed the facade was. The present owners have kept the building in an excellent state of decorations and it looks as smart now as it probably did when it first opened.
Elevations: Ashby Ball

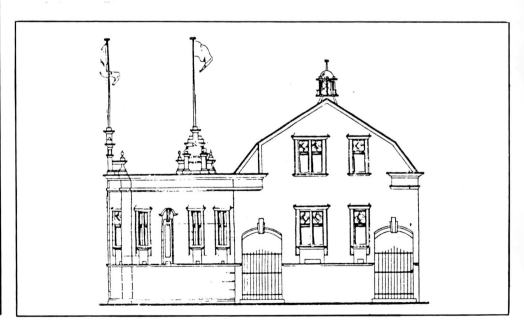

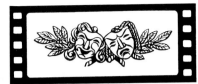

A staff outing about to leave the cinema.
Photo: *Southport Visitor*

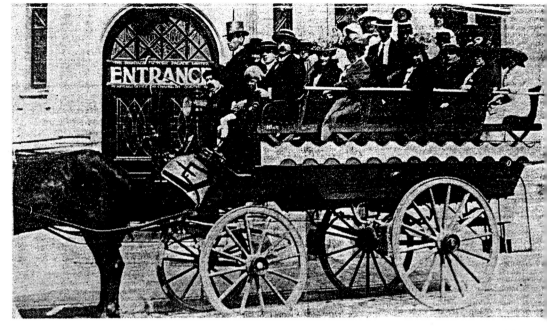

The first talkie made in Britain, *Blackmail*, is showing at the Birkdale Picture Palace. Lack of sound proofing spelled the end of the cinema and it closed in the early 1930's.
Photo: Mrs. P. Wright

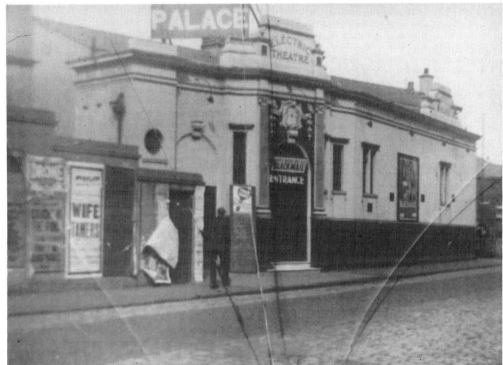

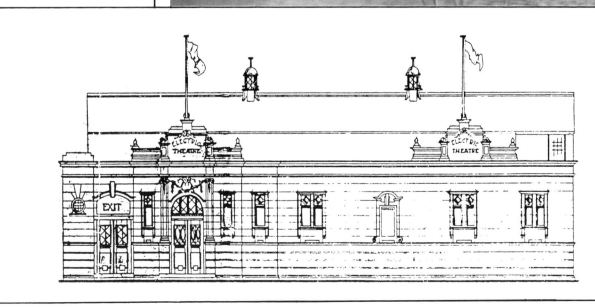

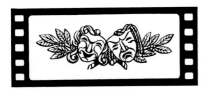

"The World Before Your Eyes" is promised. This programme dates from 1914.

Playbill: Cedric Greenwood, *Southport Visitor*

BIRKDALE PICTURE PALACE

UPPER AUGHTON ROAD AND MOSLEY STREET

| Manager | ... | ... | ... | ... | ... | ... | ... | Mr. A. Wade |
| Proprietors | | ... | ... | ... | | THE BIRKDALE PICTURE PALACE CO. LTD. | | |

The WORLD BEFORE YOUR EYES ENTERTAINMENT.

Entire Change of PROGRAMME every
MONDAY, THURSDAY, and SUNDAY.

DAILY PERFORMANCES:

First House	...	...	7 p.m.
Second House	...	...	9 p.m.
Sunday	...	...	8-15 p.m.

MATINEES:

Saturday, and Tuesday ... 3 p.m.

PRICES OF ADMISSION:

FIRST STALLS,	SECOND STALLS,	PIT,
9d. & 6d.	4d.	3d.

Children Half-price to Stalls only.
MATINEES:

| 6d. | 4d. | 2d. |

Seats booked by Telephone must be paid for before the commencement of the performance or will be sold.

Patrons will oblige by reporting any complaint to the Manager.

The Management reserve the right to refuse admission.

Box Office open, 10 to 12 and 4 to 8.

Telephone: Birkdale 438

Tel. Hours: 10-0 to 12-0 a.m. 4-0 to 6-0 p.m.

Sundays, 7 to 8

PROGRAMME FREE.

NOTICE.—The Proprietors of the above Picture Theatre have spared no expense in beautifully Decorating and Upholstering: therefore making it one of the cosiest and up-to-date Picture Theatres in Lancashire. The Pictures are the best produced and the comfort and orderliness is pronounced.

During the twenties there was a change of management to Mr W.J. Speakman, who in later years was the managing director of a circuit of cinemas in the North-West, also three times chairman of the north-western branch of the Cinematograph Exhibitors' Association.

This being one of the cinemas in the Southport area which in later years had no press advertisements, and in the absence of any recorded information, the closing date of the cinema cannot be stated. However, it appears to have survived to show the "talkies" in the early thirties, since this resulted in a petition for its closure by local residents, who complained about the noise emanating from the building, which was not soundproofed. The petition was successful and put an end to the short history of what was described as a happy institution.

After nearly forty years of oblivion and a period as a confectionery warehouse for White Hudson Ltd., memories of the old Birkdale Picture Palace were revived in 1976 when film posters adorned the walls of the auditorium, interspersed between posters for modern racing cycles. The film posters were found in the loft while central heating was being installed for the new cycle store, which was opened by Mr Jack Massey and his son, Peter, and brought back memories for many elderly local residents, who recalled going to the pictures there in the days of silent movies.

Despite another change of use in the 1980s to a light industrial workshop, many of the principal features of the auditorium are still to be seen.

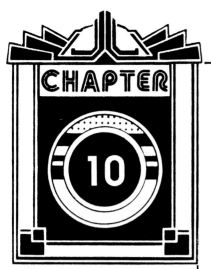

CHAPTER 10

The Palladium, built in a free Italian Renaissance style, was enhanced by its position in Lord Street, with gardens and a fountain in front of it, 1914.
Photo: C. Cramp

Following pages:
Page 51: A similar view to the one below taken a few years later. Notice the amount of advertising which now covers the cinema.
Page 52: 3rd January 1915, one year after opening. An army of over 30 staff looked after the Palladium when wages were low.
Photos: Ken Lloyd

PALLADIUM/GAUMONT/ODEON, Lord Street, Southport

The site of the Palladium was formerly occupied by a large Victorian villa, Haughton House, and a pair of semi-detached houses, which had the architectural feature of arcading on the ground floor, a style which was adopted by architect George E. Tonge for the Palladium Theatre. The houses were demolished in the spring of 1913 and construction of the theatre was commenced by T.A. Halliwell, a Southport stonemason who built the Monument and many of the town's banks.

In the free Italian Renaissance style, the building had an imposing frontage of Darley Dale stone and consisted of a principal centre section flanked on either side by a tower with segmental pediments in the cornice and pilasters extending up to the coping. Between the towers at the head of a flight of stone steps, five archways led into the arcaded portico with a line of doors to the foyer. Above the portico the colonnaded balcony had direct access from the first floor cafe, whilst a feature of the upper part of the frontage was a balustraded parapet with a row of lamp standards according with the style of the ornamental gardens laid by the Southport corporation in front of the theatre.

The spacious foyer measuring approximately 50ft. by 30ft. had a vaulted ceiling supported by columns, there was a pay-box at either side and between these a white marble staircase led to right and left up to the first floor with entrances to the Grand Circle and cafe. The latter was a luxurious room with Corinthian pillars and walls and ceiling designed in the style of the Adam period with many reproductions of original ornaments. The decoration was in soft shades of Wedgwood, the predominant colour was pale greyish-blue. Wide corridors led to the curved fronted balcony with domed boxes in the 1,500 seat auditorium decorated in the style of the English 18th century with an elliptical ceiling of exceptionally graceful lines supported on a decorated frieze beneath which were attractive pilasters. The colour scheme was of grey, cream and white enriched with gold, whilst all the draperies and carpets were of rose colour.

The stage, which had been designed for dramatic and operatic productions was 56ft. wide and 40ft. deep, and separated from the auditorium by a fireproof screen. The

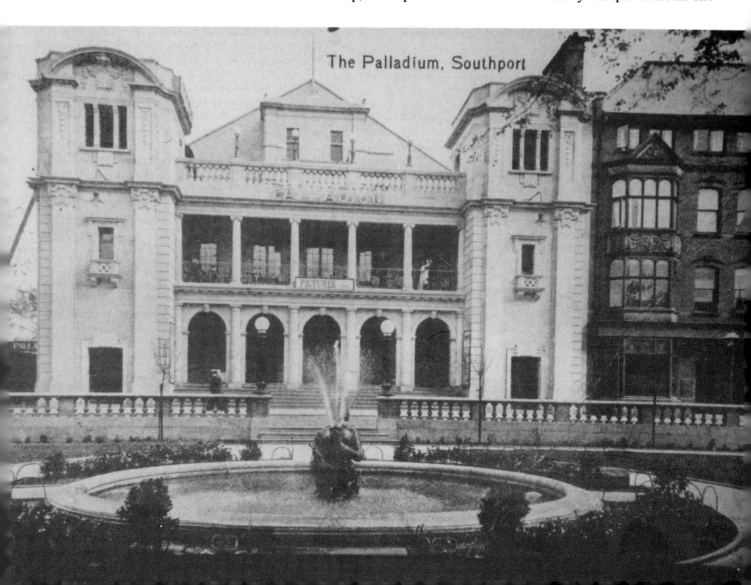

The Palladium, Southport

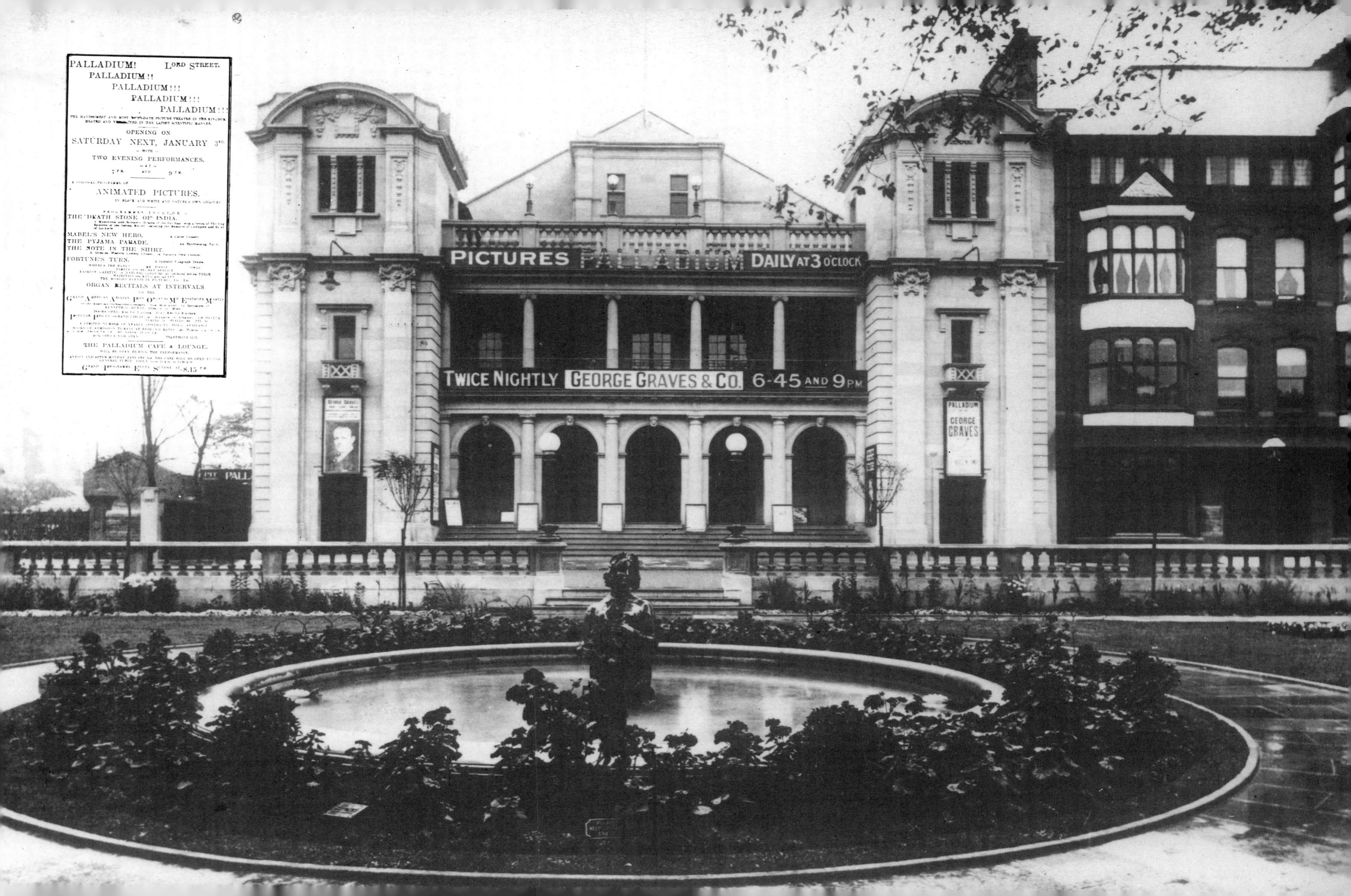

PICTURES PALLADIUM DAILY AT 3 O'CLOCK

TWICE NIGHTLY GEORGE GRAVES & CO. 6-45 AND 9 PM

GEORGE GRAVES

PALLADIUM

PALLADIUM! LORD STREET.
PALLADIUM!!
PALLADIUM!!!
PALLADIUM!!!!

OPENING ON

SATURDAY NEXT, JANUARY 3RD

TWO EVENING PERFORMANCES.
7 P.M. AND 9 P.M.

ANIMATED PICTURES.

ORGAN RECITALS AT INTERVALS

THE PALLADIUM CAFE & LOUNGE.

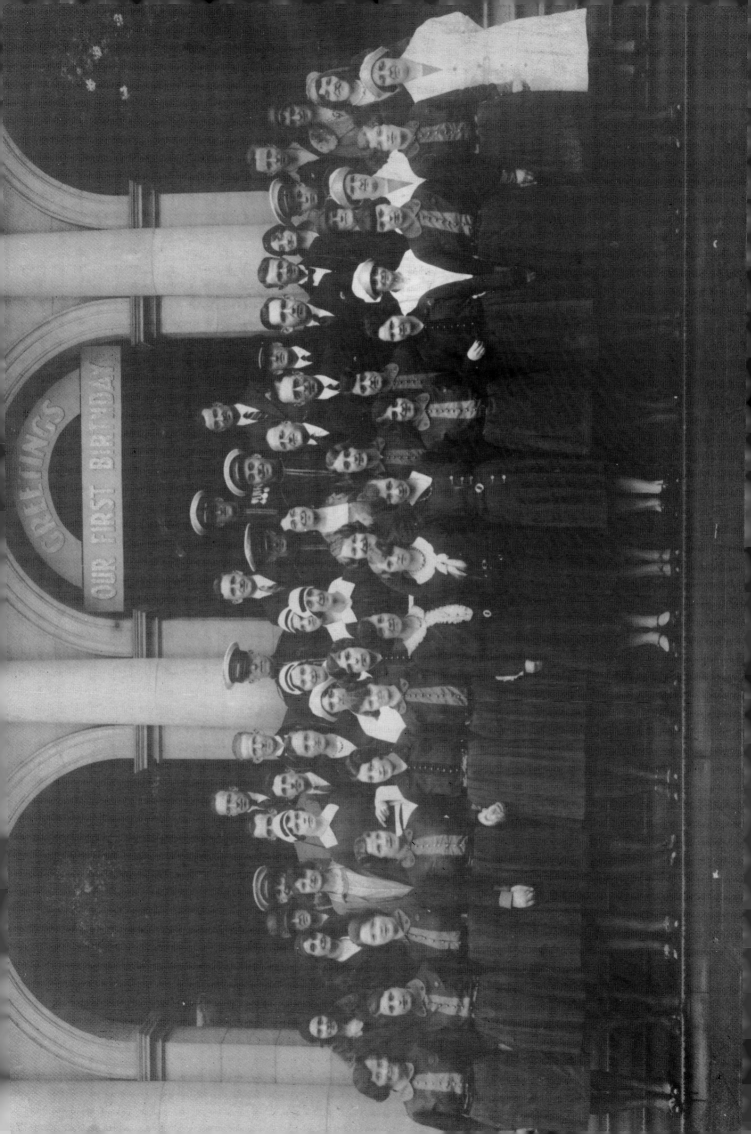

GREETINGS

OUR FIRST BIRTHDAY

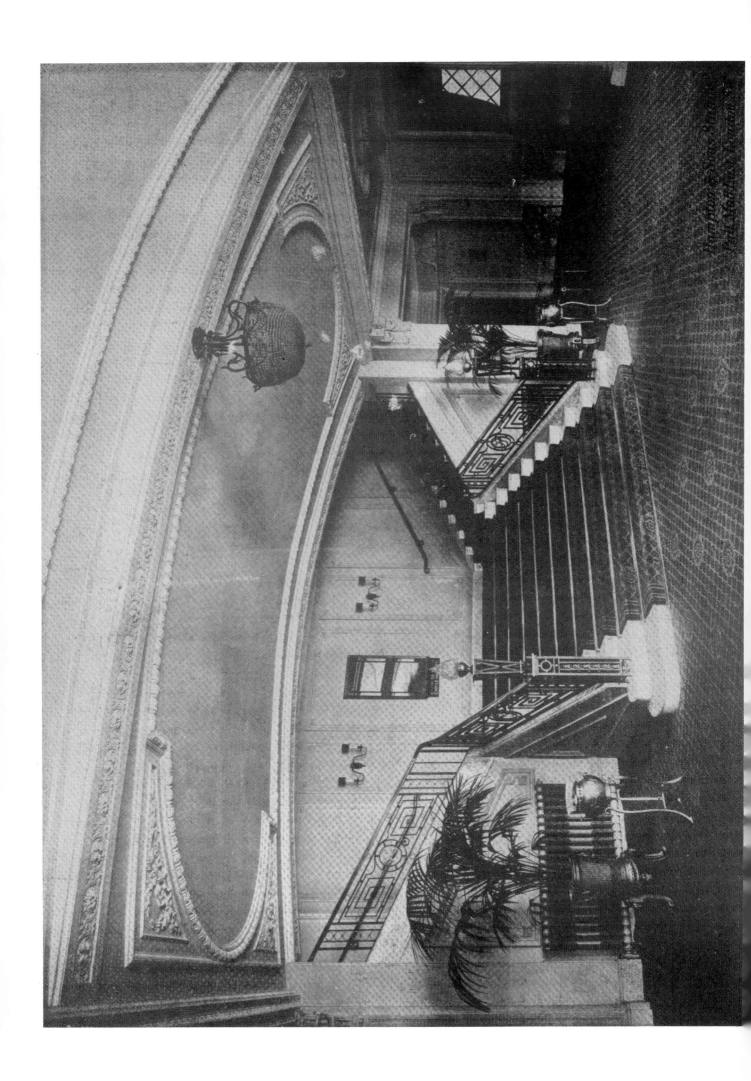

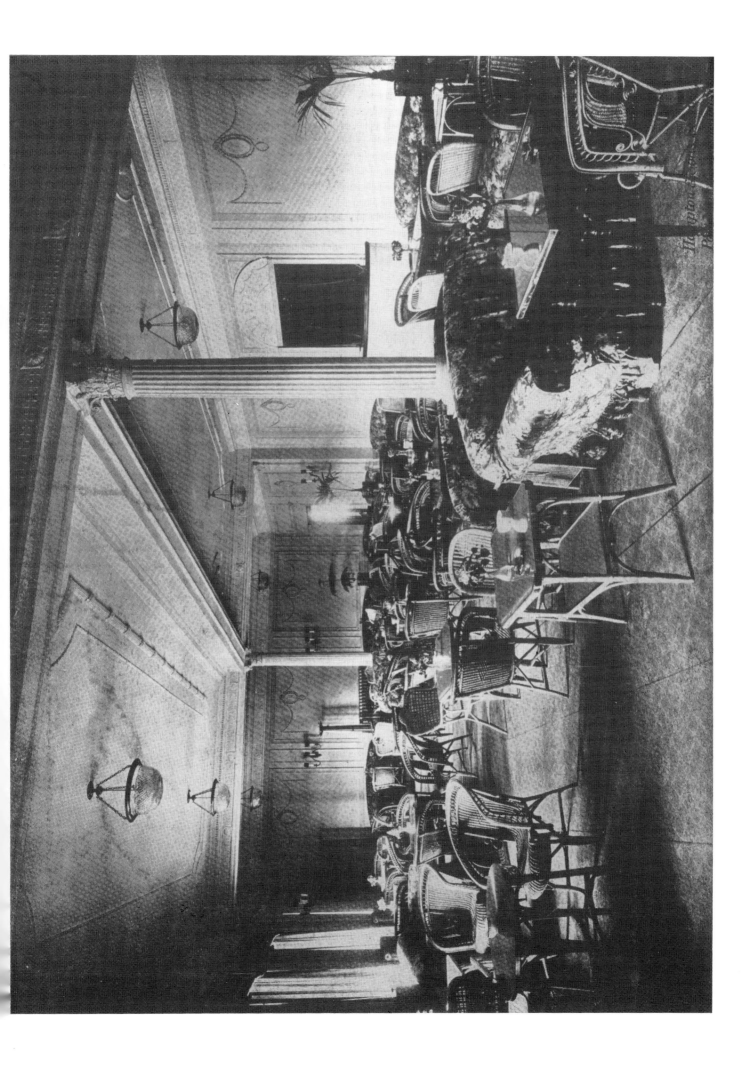

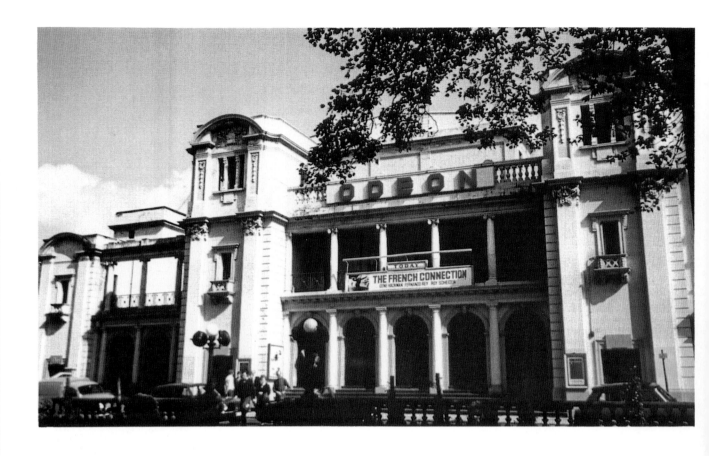

The Palladium became the Gaumont
and then the Odeon, as seen above.

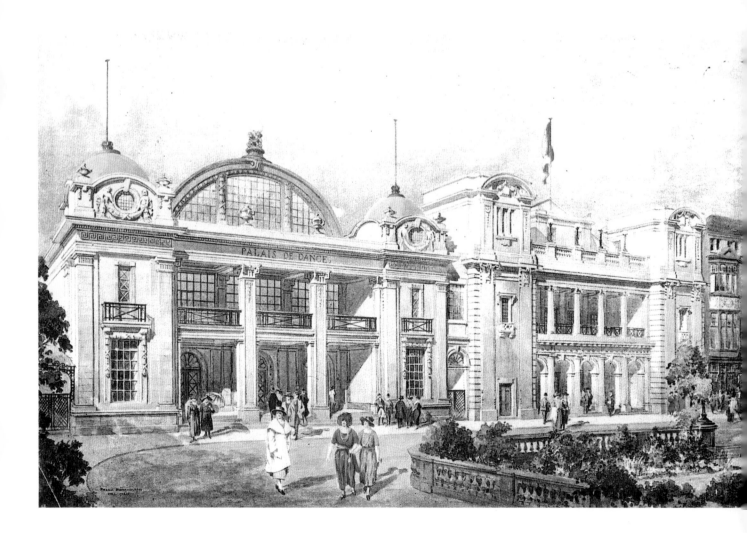

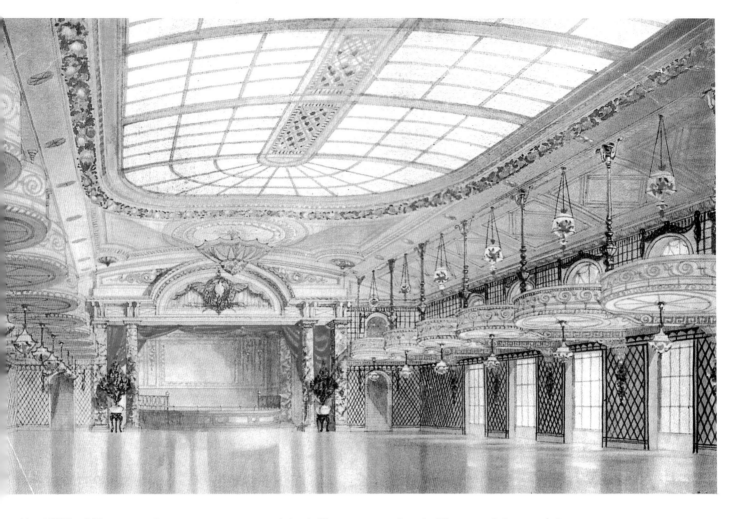

About 1926 ambitious proposals were made for a Palais de Dance adjoining the Palladium, but which were never carried out. The architect's water colour illustrations show what an asset this would have been had the proposals been carried out.
Photos: Ken Lloyd

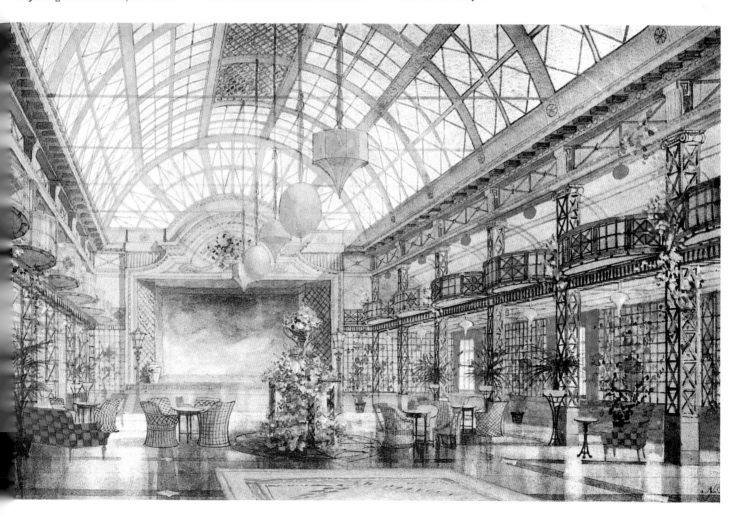

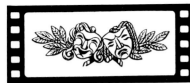

This page: The Palladium was reconstructed as the New Palladium, after a fire in 1925, although the original frontage was retained. Re-opened at Easter 1926, the New Palladium was destroyed by fire in 1929. It was again re-opened the following year as the Palladium still. It became the Gaumont in 1948.
Photo: Ken Lloyd

Following pages:
The original auditorium when opened as the Palladium. The pipes of the Aeolian organ mounted on a balcony, plus domed boxes in the circle, formed a novel and strikingly effective feature.
Photos: Ken Lloyd

SOUTHPORT GAUMONT

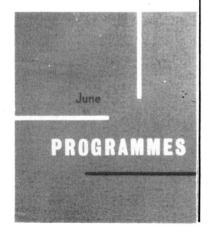

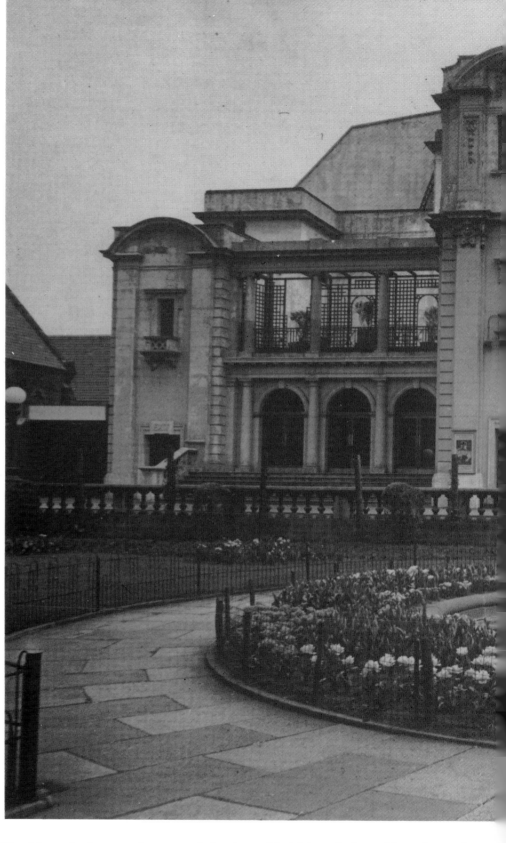

37ft. wide, arched proscenium was of about equal height, and adorned by a deep pelmet and hanging drapes of deep red rose colour with gold enrichments below which the cinema screen appeared insignificant, in the lower half of the proscenium, but accounted for by the fact that the Palladium was to be principally a theatre. A novel and strikingly effective feature of the auditorium was that along either side and terminating at the boxes were the pipes of the Aeolian organ mounted on a balcony.

The principal lighting was by elegant chandeliers suspended by chains from the ceiling, each with torch-style light fittings spaced around the edge, which greatly enhanced the bright colour scheme of the decorations.

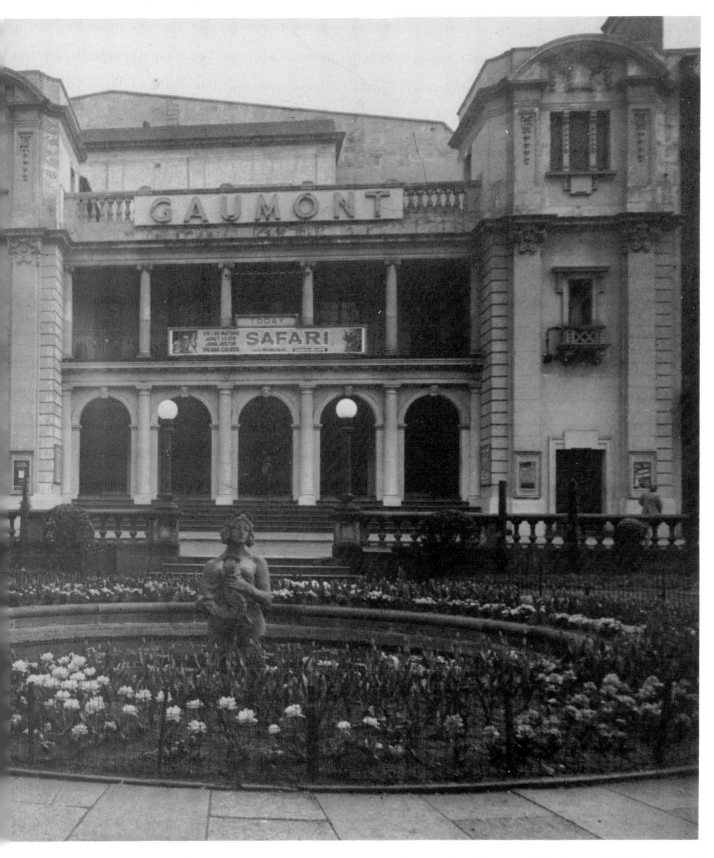

The Palladium was originally owned and operated by Leonard Williamson of Hesketh Park, Southport, and advertised as the handsomest and most up-to-date picture theatre in the U.K. The Grand Opening took place with a special invitation performance on the afternoon of 3rd January 1914, when the packed "house" included the Mayor and Mayoress, Councillor and Mrs Limont and a number of town councillors. The performance opened with an overture on the Grand American Aeolian pipe organ by Mr. Easthope Martin, then followed a supporting programme of short films entitled - *The Note in the Shirt* (handsomely coloured), *Where's the Baby?*, *Fashion Gazette* (in Nature's own colours), *The Pyjama Parade* (cartoon) and *Fortune's Turn*. After the organ interlude the feature film was *The Death Stone of India*, a mysterious and romantic drama of the far east.

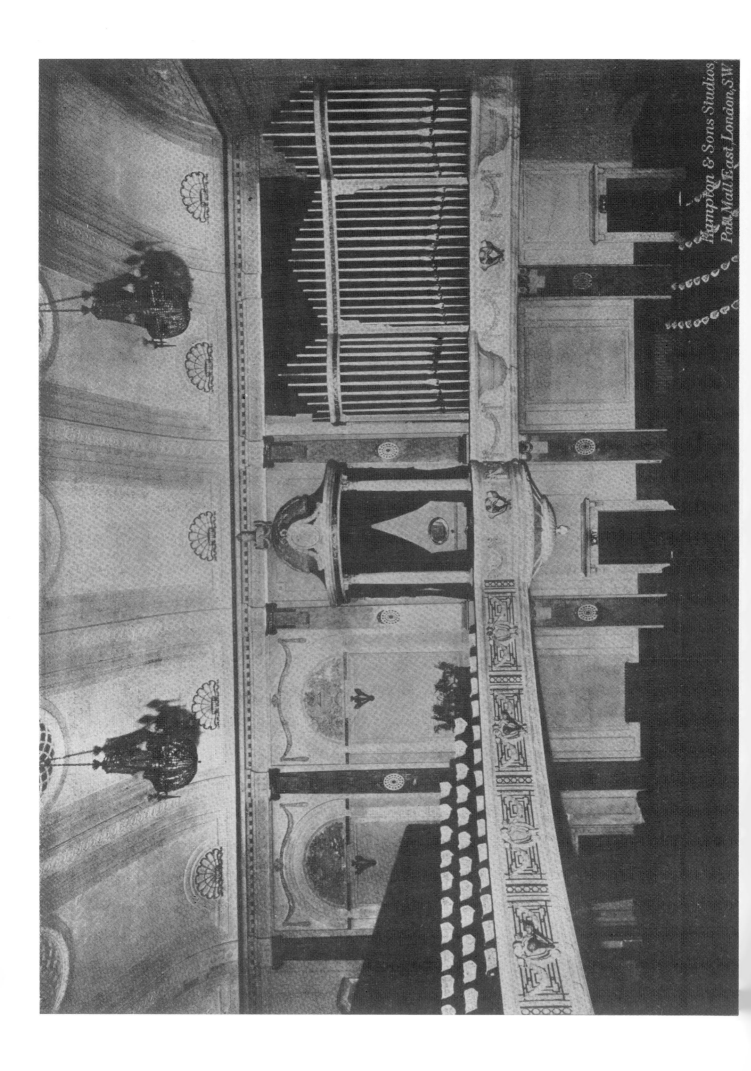

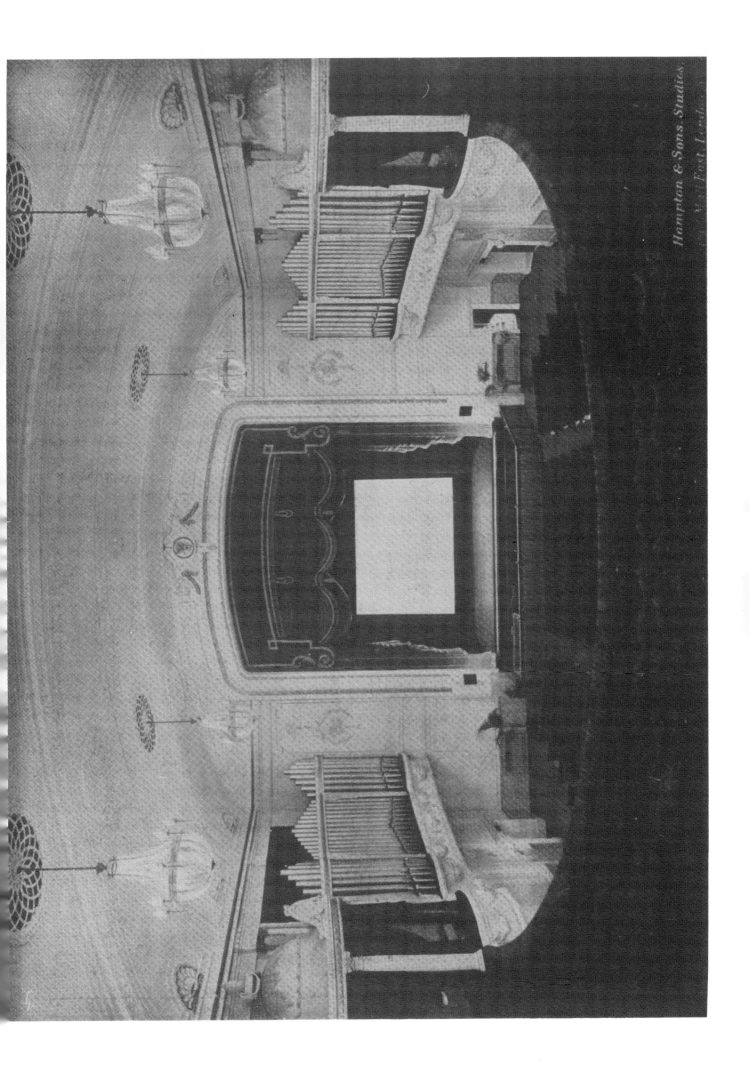

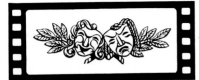

The first owner was Leonard Williamson (below) who had a policy of cine-variety. This was a programme of first class films and variety on the stage. The photo (right) shows how elaborate these stage shows were.
Photos: Ken Lloyd

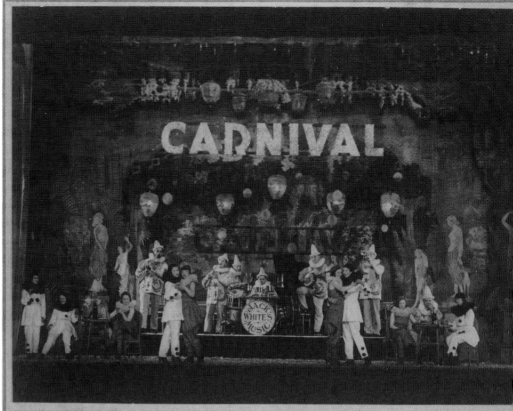

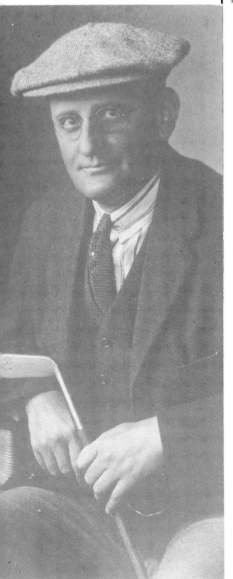

In the evening there were performances at 7pm and 9pm, but the occasion of the first public show was marred by the incident at 6.30pm when the doors opened, a tremendous crowd of people were waiting outside, of which about 600 broke loose from the middle of the queue and rushed up the steps and into the foyer to the pay-boxes. The crowd became quickly out of control and the police had to be called to restore order! With the police still in attendance no further trouble was experienced from another large crowd for the second house at 9pm.

Patrons paid 2/- for a seat in the circle (bookable in advance) whilst the orchestra stalls were 1/-, the stalls 6d and the pit 3d. The cafe was open during the performances on the day of opening and thereafter from 11am to 10.30pm.

Although the Palladium opened with films, thereafter these were confined to Sundays, the artistes' day of rest, the remainder of the week being allocated to 'live' entertainment with music by a resident orchestra in addition to the organ, and among the many famous artistes who appeared there were George Formby senior, Marie Lloyd, Hetty King, Ella Shields, Little Tich, and Southport's own male impersonator, and dancer, Rosie Walmsley.

Leonard Williamson's reign was succeeded in 1921 by Southport Palladium Ltd. of which the managing director was John L. Dixon who maintained a programme policy of first class films and variety on the stage with Herbert Steele, the theatre's musical director at the organ. This terminated on 20th October 1925 due to a serious fire in the auditorium during the early hours, when although the fire was confined by the fire brigade to a portion of the dress circle, the seats, carpeting and decorations in other parts of the theatre were considerably damaged by many gallons of water at a cost of several thousand pounds. During the next five months, Southport architects, Gray & Evans co-operated with Mr. Dixon in the work of restoration, producing what was described as a masterpiece among picture houses. It was stated that the architectural beauty of the building had been accentuated, starting with the entrance hall where the ceiling in blue and the walls blending from russet to cream with gilded plaster ornamentation served as a fitting introduction to the magnificence of the auditorium. Therein the wall panelling was in blended colouring and the ceiling panelled in soft blue embellished with gold stars and mouldings in matching tints with gilded enrichments. The draperies, seating and carpets were in purple, whilst the silk shades on the chandeliers and the special lighting effects were admirable features. The stage was widened by about 13ft. and a new proscenium arch constructed so that an uninterrupted view of the entire stage could be obtained from every seat in the house including the side seats on the front row. Surviving the fire, the organ was throughly overhauled and restored to its original high standard.

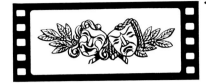

The most important event of Easter 1926 was the re-opening of the theatre, then to be known as the New Palladium at 6.15pm on 3rd April when a large audience was enthusiastic about the wondrous improvements which had been made. The special programme for the day of the world's finest productions was headed by the feature film *Siege* featuring Virginia Valli, with supporting programme including the latest news on *Pathe Super Gazette*. Seats in the Grand Circle were reduced from 1/6d to 1/3d whilst the stalls remained at 6d and 1/-.Following the opening there were three performances each weekday at 3pm, 6.30pm and 8.40pm.

The former policy of cine-variety was re-instated and the theatre continued under the ownership of Southport Palladium Ltd. until 1928, when following rumours for several weeks that negotiations for the sale of the building were in progress, the local press, *Southport Visitor* on 25th February reported the announcement that the theatre had been acquired by a London syndicate controlled by Sir Walter Gibbons and the great financier, F.A.Szarvasy, in a major deal which also included 13 Merseyside halls then coming under the control of the company known as the General Theatres Corporation Ltd. Mr. Will Hughes, who had a long association with Southport entertainments dating back over 15 years to his time at the Winter Gardens, was appointed general manager of the Palladium, the word New having been dispensed with. Announcing startling innovations, Mr. Hughes stated his aim to enhance the comfort of patrons and provide the very best in pictures and music, and with regard to the latter he was fortunate to secure the services of Harold Gee and his orchestra, in addition to retaining Herbert Steele as the theatre's musical director and organist, both of whom were included in the programmes from Easter Monday 1928. Another new innovation was the policy for the first time in Southport of continuous performances, Monday to Friday from 6.30pm to 10.45 pm, and two separate shows on Saturdays only at 6.30pm and 8.40pm. To all evening performances there was one price to the stalls at 9d, whilst seats in the circle were 1/3d and 2/-. Bargain matinees at 2.45pm Monday to Saturday were introduced with admission to the entire ground floor, 1,000 seats at 6d.

Adding to the attractions of the theatre only two years after the many improvements, the new innovations were most successful and attracted record crowds. It was therefore extremely unfortunate that it all came to an end with another far more widespread fire than that of 1925, for on the night of 26th March 1929, the auditorium was burnt out, leaving the frontage including the foyer and the cafe the only surviving parts of the building. To have rebuilt the Palladium on similar lines would have been a comparatively easy matter, but fine as the old building had undoubtedly been, the directors of the General Theatres

The Compton organ rose to stage level on a lift in the centre of the orchestra pit. This was a popular feature of the rebuilt Palladium of 1930.
Photo: John Sharp

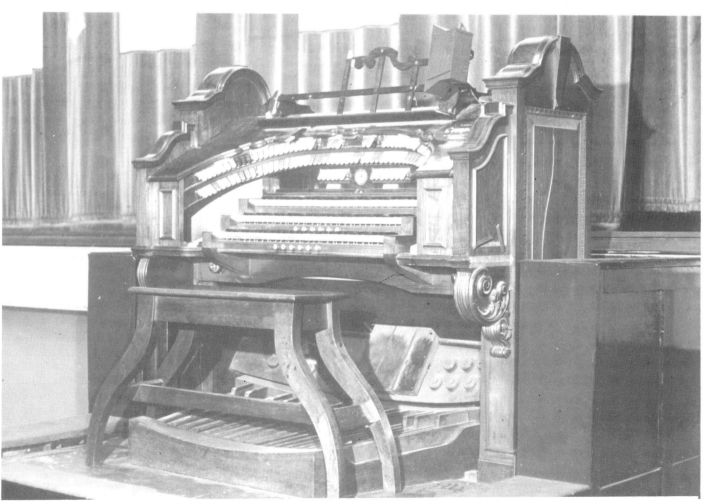

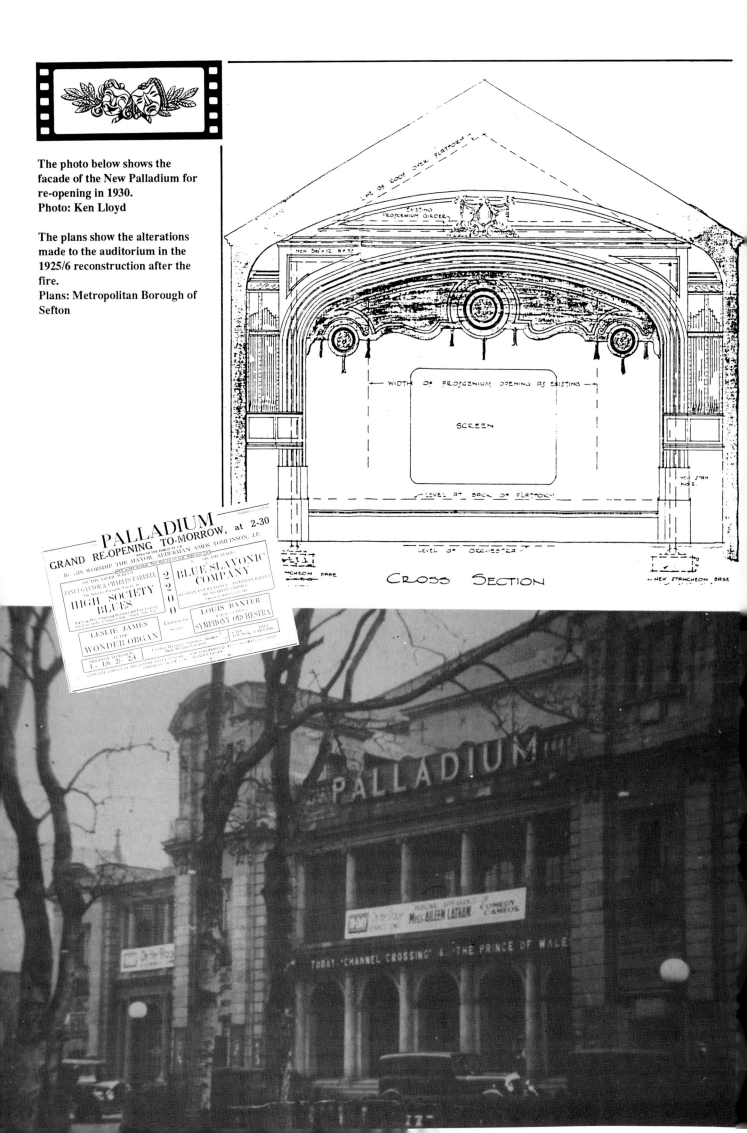

The photo below shows the
facade of the New Palladium for
re-opening in 1930.
Photo: Ken Lloyd

The plans show the alterations
made to the auditorium in the
1925/6 reconstruction after the
fire.
Plans: Metropolitan Borough of
Sefton

CROSS SECTION

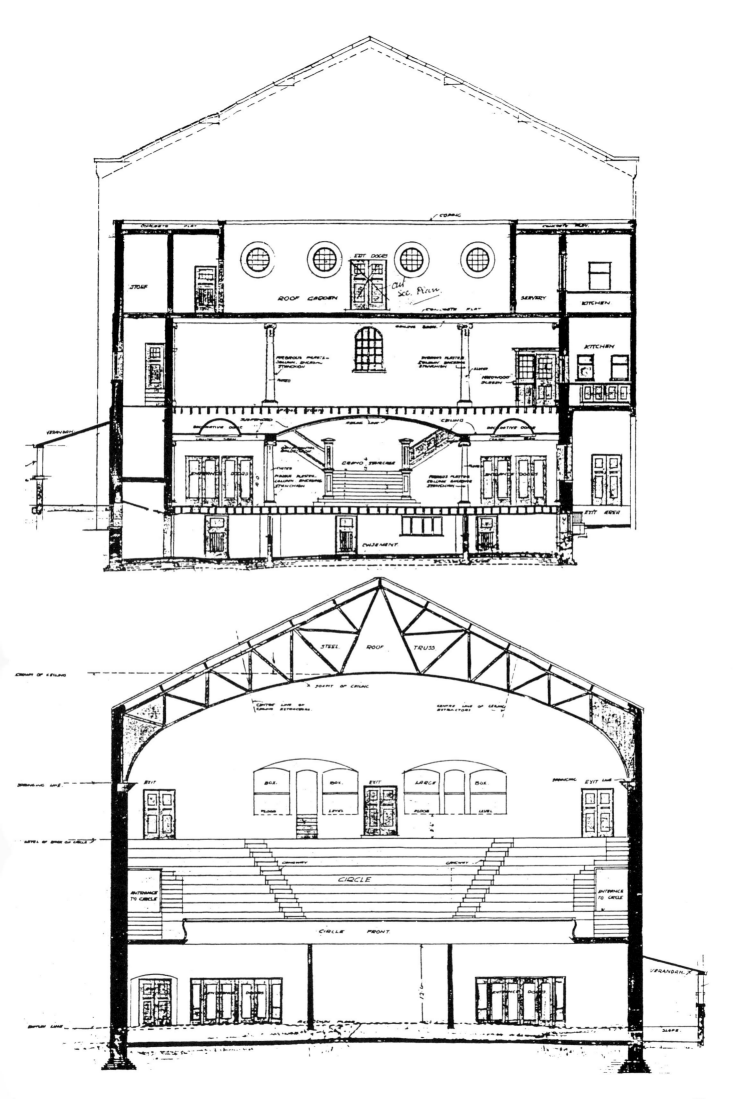

65

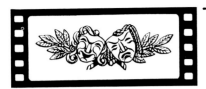

Opposite and following pages:
A 1928 programme for the Palladium is described as a G.T.C. Theatre, a subsidiary of Gaumont British. This shows that they already owned the Palladium before the disastrous fire and did not buy the site afterwards as is generally thought.
Programme: Ken Lloyd

Corporation in association with the Gaumont British Picture Corporation decided on the construction of an even finer theatre from every point of view - size, decoration, comfort, and with the march of progress in the film world - future entertainment.

The architect, W.E. Trent, FSI designed a new theatre almost double the width of the old, made possible by the fortunate possession of spare land at the left hand side. The original frontage had therefore to be extended accordingly, and the new elevation made subsidiary to it so that the impressiveness of the two flanking towers should not be lost. The same details of archways, columns and cornices were followed, and at first floor level an open colonnade was filled in with trellis work for the display of flowers and creepers during the summer in harmony with the gardens of Lord Street.

The flight of stone steps in the original entrance and the matching extension gave access via a line of doors, including in the former, a central revolving door to the foyer of which the width had been increased to 96ft. This had a marble mosaic floor, enriched plaster ceiling, wood lined walls and square columns, stained a pale grey matching the grey, green and silver of the ceiling. From the foyer a short flight of steps in the centre leading to two pairs of doors to the rear of the stalls,was flanked by two staircases to the first floor where the restaurant and waiting room retained the Wedgwood style of decoration. Corridors led to the entrances at either side of the balcony with accommodation for about 700 in the 2,200 seat auditorium, which conveyed a feeling of great space and airiness due to the wide, curved sweep of the balcony across the width of 120ft. Forward of the balcony front, long splayed walls incorporating the organ grilles extended to the 52ft. wide proscenium, set within a curved area, illuminated in various colours by concealed lighting. In addition to films it was intended that stage shows and revues should continue to form an important part of the entertainment, and providing for this the stage was 30ft. deep with 22 lines of backdrops and spacious dressing room accommodation was included at the rear. Although to re-open as a Talkie Theatre, music was nevertheless still considered of great importance, a large orchestra pit being constructed in front of the stage, with a lift in the centre upon which was installed the latest Compton organ rising to stage level. This replaced the Aeolian pipe organ which had been such a popular feature of the old theatre.

The decorative treatment was unconventional, being in horizontal bands of deep blue, green and red plush, separated by silver lines above a dado of polished walnut. The entire scheme was enhanced by the varied tints of the concealed lighting, a special feature of which was installed in the trough at the base of the large dome above the balcony, whilst the principal illumination was provided by long, straight sided glass-shaded fittings suspended from the ceiling. The seats were stated to be the last word in comfort, of the standard type used by Gaumont British with excellent sight lines to the stage and screen, the rear half of the stalls as those in the circle being on a stepped floor. Opening at a time of the growing popularity of the "talkies" the Palladium was equipped with British Acoustics sound system, and a wide screen enabling everyone to see the picture with the greatest ease. Since music was to form an important part of the entertainment, in addition to the Compton organ an orchestra of 20 musicians was engaged.

The Grand Re-opening of the Palladium at 2.30pm on 1st October 1930 was by His Worship the Mayor of Southport, Alderman Amos Tomlinson J.P. accompanied by a representative group of townspeople. The film programme opened with *British Movietone News*, followed by *Roman Punch* and a Terry Toon cartoon. Then, on the stage, The Blue Slavonic Dance Company gave an exhibition of Russian and Hungarian Court and Gypsy dances. Music was provided by Louis Baxter and his famous symphony orchestra, and organ interludes by Leslie James before the feature film *High Society Blues* featuring Janet Gaynor and Charles Farrell. The Palladium was the first cinema theatre in Southport to run performances continuous from 2pm to 10.30pm except for Sunday which was still restricted to one performance at 8.15pm. Prices of admission at the opening were 1/-, 1/ 6d, 2/- and 2/4d. Herbert Steele, who had been the theatre's musical director and resident organist through the 1920s until the fire, returned to play the organ from 6th October 1930. Retiring in 1939 he was succeeded by Cecil Williams (real name William Hopper) from the Gaumont, Chester, who continued as the organist until 1942.

Although opened as a cine-variety theatre, the resident orchestra soon proved too costly to maintain, resulting in the end of "live" entertainment in January 1931, but the new organ, rising and falling on the lift for the intervals continued to be a popular added attraction to the film programmes. The Gaumont and Odeon circuits amalgamated in 1947, and in accordance with the company policy the theatre was renamed the Gaumont.

Although ideally suited to CinemaScope, copyrighted by Twentieth Century Fox in 1953, probably as a result of the producer's dispute with the Rank Organisation in 1954.

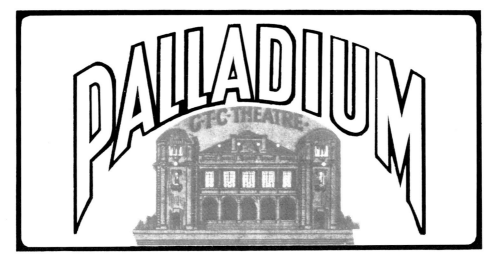

THE MOST POPULAR HOUSE IN SOUTHPORT.

ENORMOUS SUCCESS of

HAROLD GEE

AND HIS

ALL BRITISH ORCHESTRA.

Greeted by Thunderous Applause at Every Performance. Acclaimed by Press and Public as the Greatest Combination of Musicians ever presented in any Cinema in Southport.

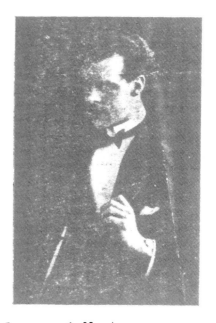

A Real Delight to Southport Lovers of Music.

AT EVERY PERFORMANCE, *including*—

6d. BARGAIN MATINEES **6d.**

DIUM
HEATRE.

... ... Mr. WILL HUGHES.

❋❋❋❋❋❋❋❋❋❋❋❋❋❋❋❋❋❋❋❋❋❋❋❋❋❋❋❋

AMME ::
AY, APRIL 16th, 1928

THURSDAY, FRIDAY, & SATURDAY

Pathe Gazette............All the Latest Topical Events

Screaming ....Comedy

On the Stage.

Victor Bright & Luna Denver
Present
"NAUTICALITIS"

Eve's Review ....Interesting Tit-Bits

Musical Interlude by
HAROLD GEE
and his All British Orchestra.

JETTA GOUDAL in
WHITE GOLD

He took her from a pleasant life, to a lonely existence on the burning plains. She gave up all for his love---and when it failed her . . . . !

m.   Two Super Pictures.

WRATH OF THE GODS."
AMOUS WONDER ORGAN.

NOTE—
SATURDAYS TWO DISTINCT PERFORMANCES
AT 6-40 AND 8-50 P.M.
SEATS MAY BE BOOKED IN ADVANCE.
Balcony 1/6.   Stalls 1/-
Including Tax and Booking Fee.
Box Office Open from 10 a.m.

NEXT WEEK.

ON THE SCREEN.

Thursday to Saturday.

The Rival Picture to 'Beau Geste'

CONRAD VEIDT

IN

A Man's Past

Conrad Veidt as the sorrow sodden convict. His acting is the profoundest piece of work ever seen—a masterpiece of screen acting that will never be surpassed.

ON THE STAGE.
LONDON'S FAVOURITE
RUSSELL CARR
VENTRILOQUIST
Assisted by OLIVE GRAY.

WHEN IN LIVERPOOL, VISIT
RIALTO BALLROOM
The Acme of Perfection and Refinement.

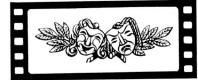

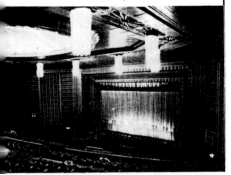

The Wurlitzer organ was a popular feature of the Gaumont as the photos taken in the 1930s show. The photo below shows the auditorium as rebuilt by W.E. Trent in 1930. The photo at the bottom shows Stanley Harrison at the organ and the one bottom right shows Herbert Steele, organist and musical director
Photos: John Sharp

there was considerable delay in equipping the Gaumont where CinemaScope opened on 26th October 1954 with the Universal picture *The Black Shield of Falworth* featuring Tony Curtis. The entire projection equipment was renewed by G.B. Kalee Ltd. with a time limit of 18 hours after the last performance on 19th January 1957, when G.B. Kalee 21 projectors, arcs and sound equipment were installed. This coincided with the equipping, also by G.B. Kalee of the Garrick Theatre as a cinema.

The period from 1955 to 1964 can justifiably be considered the theatre's greatest era as the Gaumont, under the management of Mr Kenneth Lloyd one of Rank's leading showmen. "Live" entertainment was re-introduced, apparently for the first time since 1931 with one-night big-name shows, as now staged at the Southport Theatre. Unprecedented scenes and fantastic business resulted from three visits of the Beatles during the height of Beatlemania in the early sixties, and others who starred there included Cyril Stapleton and his band, Cliff Richard, Helen Shapiro, Marion Ryan, Ronnie Hilton and Gerry & The Pacemakers.

Mr William Hopper, the former organist, returned as assistant manager, also playing the organ until 1964, the instrument having survived thanks to Mr Lloyd, despite Rank's bid to remove it in 1963. Further organ interludes in the mid-sixties were by Mr Charles Smart, and prior to being removed in the early seventies. The organ was last played by the manager, Mr Laurie Hindmarsh who revived organ recitals at Sunday afternoon shows in 1971/2.

The decline of the theatre, renamed the Odeon in 1962, began about the mid-sixties, by which time "live" entertainment had ceased, and the cafe was closed. The theatre had been described as a "Cathedral of the Movies" but as such, in its later years, it dwarfed the dwindling congregation of the faithful few. There was speculation about conversion into a bowling centre, then a bingo hall, but both schemes were resisted and films continued in the huge single screen cinema, although from 1974 with performances normally restricted to evenings, and matinees on Thursday and Saturday only.

With the Odeon still running at a loss, the Rank Organisation suddenly announced closure on 22nd November 1975, but reconsidered and decided to continue the restricted operation, with some limited improvements hoping to boost the profitability of the theatre. Internally, the oil fired central heating system was improved whilst the flaking surface of the facade was treated with masonry paint resistant to salty air.

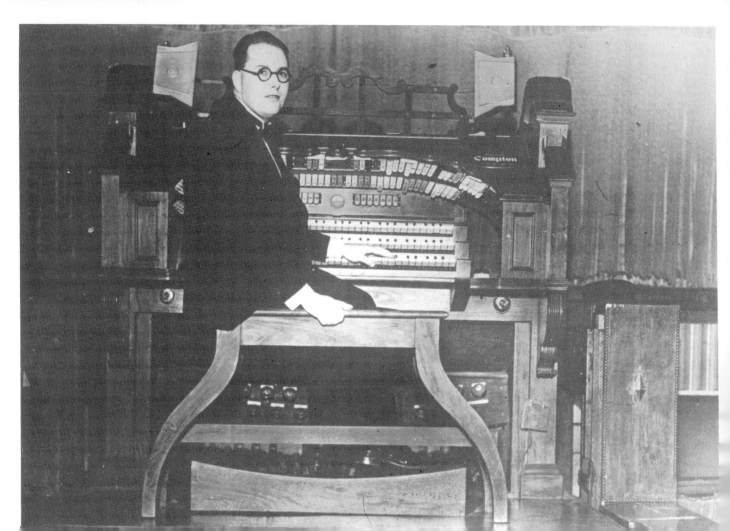

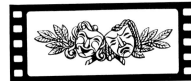

The Odeon, as the cinema finally became in 1962, was never tripled, unlike many large cinemas during the 1970's.
Photo: Mike Taylor

The newspaper advert for the Odeon is interesting, not so much for the films being shown, but for the live show. A total of six top groups and singers were to be seen in the one show.
Advert: *Southport Journal*, Wednesday 10th July 1963

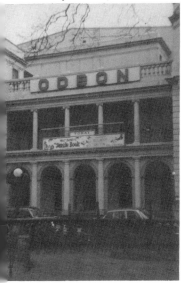

In 1979 the London grocers, J. Sainsbury Ltd. made application to the borough council for demolition of the building, and replacement with a new supermarket on the site. The case for demolition was based on a survey report which alleged that the condition of the building was poor and could not be satisfactorily restored. This did not appear to be the case, especially with regard to the original Darley Dale stone frontage, whilst the brickwork was subsequently found to have been very well maintained. The matter was the subject of a thorough investigation by the borough council, for not only was the Odeon a listed building but also had the protection of being in a conservation area. Despite this however, the developers won the case and the Rank Organisation arranged the closure for 1st December 1979 when a small audience attended for the final programme - *Confessions of a Pop Performer* and *A Game for Vultures*.

In the summer of 1980, probably few citizens - still less the developers and their contractors realised that they were demolishing the building which had been Southport's hall of fame, in which since 1914 the roll of artistes who appeared there read like a *Who's Who* and a *Who Was Who* in the world of entertainment.

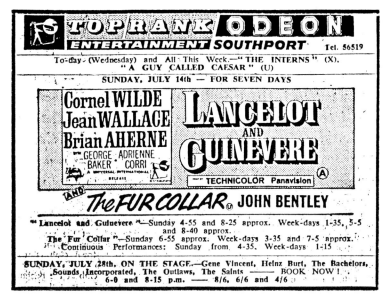

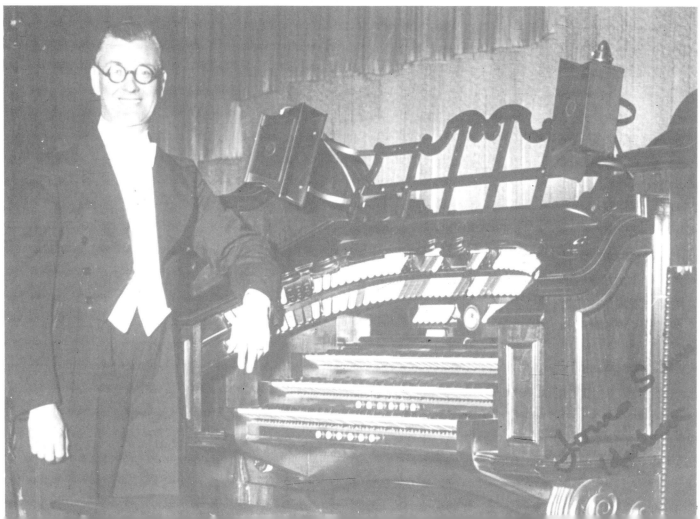

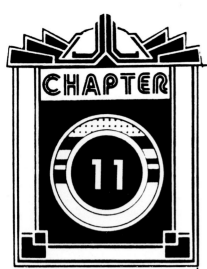

PLAZA CINEMA, BALLROOM & CAFE, Liverpool Road, Ainsdale

Erected in 1927 to the plans of Southport architect, Mr George E. Tonge, Lic. RIBA in association with Mr Felix Holt, ARIBA Liverpool, at a cost of about £15,000, the building combined a 650 seat cinema, a small ballroom, lounges and a cafe, also four shops along the frontage. The main road site, about two miles from Southport was chosen as the most suitable since future extensions of the borough were to bring the situation almost to its centre. Designed in the free Italian Renaissance style the construction was of two almost separate elevations, the frontage and the auditorium, both lengthwise to the road, with the latter angled back towards the right-hand, stage end. The two elevations were linked at ground level by the foyer extending from the central main entrance, flanked on either side by two shops. The ornamental frontage had a covering of Atlas white cement to resemble Portland stone, and a roof of red tiles, above which, in the centre the square tower was an imposing architectural feature. Below this at ground level, the main entrance was surmounted by a small canopy, whilst the ballroom extended along the first floor of the frontage.

The entrance, with two pairs of doors inset, gave access to the foyer with the pay-box immediately adjacent to the wall on the left side, beyond which, at a width of about 12ft. it extended diagonally to the right. The flooring was of coloured linoleum, decoration of the walls by panels above a "Marblequa" (marble substitute) dado and the scheme also included four fibrous plaster Corinthian columns. At the end of the foyer, entrance doors led to the right-hand side of the stadium-type auditorium about midway between the stage and rear, where a crossover gangway divided the seating into two almost equal sections. The front half was on a raked floor whilst the rear part was stepped, thereby providing an excellent view of the screen from all parts of the house. There was also a central gangway, and to facilitate the rapid clearing of the audience in an emergency, an exit at either side of the stage and two at the rear of the auditorium. The seats, claimed to be the last word in style and comfort were of the semi-tub type resembling an easy chair, the covering was of royal blue mohair velvet and the woodwork of polished mahogany. Fitted at a distance of nearly 3ft. between each row, patrons could pass along without disturbing those seated. Adding further to the comfort, the entire floor was covered by carpet.

Features of the decorations, treated in an Eastern style, were the "Marblequa" pillars, pilasters and panelling carried out by the Southport firm of W.G. Crotch Ltd. whose recent work at that time was the remarkable ornamental plaster work at the Rialto, Liverpool. Pilasters along the side walls extended up to the carved cornice, from which the curved ceiling was adorned with large glass-shaded electric fittings in matching Eastern style. A stage with dressing room at the rear provided for possible 'live' entertainment, and in front of the stage the proscenium curtain was of blue velvet.

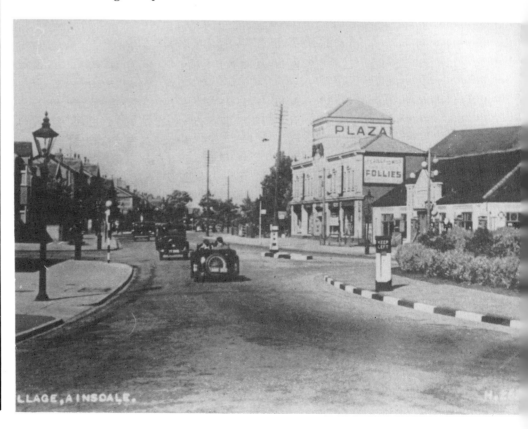

Liverpool Road presents a pastoral look as a few motor vehicles make their way past the Plaza. The photo far right clearly shows the shops either side of the main entrance. The ballroom extended across the first floor of the frontage.
Photos: D Taylor, Publicity & Attractions, Metropolitan Borough of Sefton

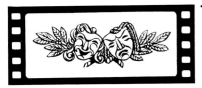

At the rear of the auditorium, between the exit ways, an extension was constructed for the projection room, equipped with Kalee 8 machines, rewinding and other associated rooms.

The first floor ballroom and cafe were approached by ascending a wide staircase from the entrance foyer to a lounge on the first floor from which doors led into the luxurious cafe, adjacent to which, the kitchen was fitted with all modern appliances. Also on this level, the ballroom had a musicians' gallery, and a special type of floor laid on buffer rubber springs, stated to have the advantage over steel springs in that the springing was noticeable only to the dancers.

Friday 27th January 1928 was considered a red letter occasion to the people of Ainsdale, for it marked the Grand Opening of the Plaza under the ownership of the Coliseum (Southport) Ltd., and considered likely to repeat the success and popularity of the Nevill Street cinema, since it was to be run on similar lines, the company having booked some very outstanding films which would be shown throughout the country. At the invitation of Mr Arnold Hadfield, chairman of the board of directors, many members of the Southport Town Council attended in the packed to capacity auditorium for the opening ceremony by the mayor, Councillor J.G. Wilkinson. During his speech from the stage Councillor Wilkinson praised the efforts of the company's managing director, Alderman Trounson, in securing for the opening an all-British production at a time of so much adverse criticism about the lack of British films. Described as probably the most thrilling film ever made, the feature film was *The Flight Commander* with Sir Alan Cobham KBE, supported by a programme of short films, all with musical accompaniment by Miss E. Ireland at the pianoforte.

With the exception of a matinee on Saturday at 2.30pm, performances were originally in the evenings only at 6.30pm and 8.50pm, but this was soon reduced to one performance Monday to Friday at 7.45pm. Admission was at 1/6d to the rear (Grand Stalls), 1/- in the centre and 6d to the front stalls. At the opening performance there was disappointment that the ballroom was not also open - surprisingly this did not take place until 3rd September 1929 when the Grand Opening was with Billy Atherton's Esmeraldo Band from the Palace Hotel. Dancing was from 8pm, admission at 1/6d.

The "talkies" having arrived at most of the town's cinemas, the silent era at the Plaza ended on 25th October 1930 with *The Doctor's Secret* starring Ruth Chatterton, also Anna Q. Nilsson in *Blockade*. B.T.P. sound system having been installed for the opening on Monday 27th October of *Sunny Side Up* featuring Janet Gaynor and Charles Farrell, also supporting programme including *British Movietone News*.

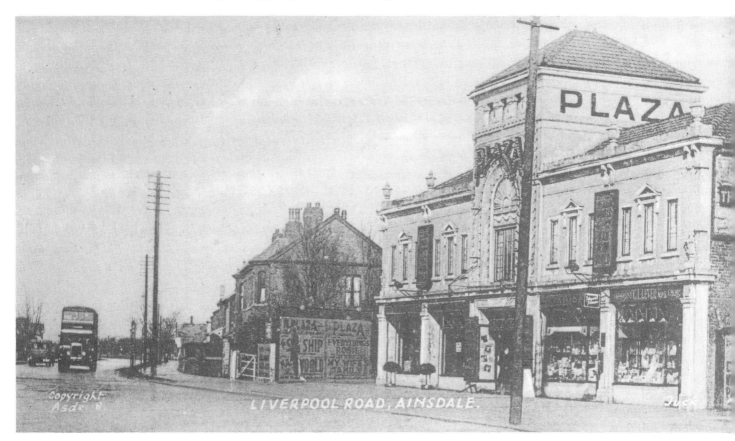

LIVERPOOL ROAD, AINSDALE.

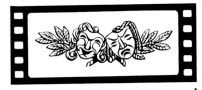

In the mid-thirties the Plaza came under the control of Associated Southport Cinemas, a company formed by the directors of Coliseum (Southport) Ltd., in association with local businessmen, Arnold Hadfield remaining as chairman of the board.

Serving a mainly local patronage, the Plaza screened films for three days only following other cinemas in the town, and in 1951 with decreasing attendances it was advertised for sale. The attention of a leisure entrepreneur and principal of the company Furness Electric Theatre Co. Ltd. was attracted, and believing he could make a success of the Plaza by continuing its use as a cinema, he acquired it, putting in hand a major scheme of refurbishment with attractive new decorations and furnishings including 600 new Dunlopillo seats in the auditorium. In addition the latest projection equipment was installed and new gas operated central heating.

Early in January 1952, large advertisements in the local press proclaimed the Plaza as Southport's latest luxury cinema offering an unequalled choice of the finest programmes including early release *Pathe News*. Four programmes weekly were to be shown with changes on Sunday, Monday, Wednesday and Friday, continuous from 6.00pm, Sunday 8.00pm.

In the summer of 1953 "The New Era in Screen Realism" was announced, the Plaza being the first cinema in the Southport area to be equipped with the latest panoramic wide screen "As installed at the Odeon, Leicester Square, London!"

But despite this latest novelty, in addition to the improvements of the previous year, the cinema continued to be sparsely attended, and in January 1957, just five years after the reopening, the Plaza was put up for sale by auction. A buyer having been found, the closing date was Saturday 11th May 1957 ending a two day showing of *It's Great to be Young* with John Mills and Cecil Parker.

The building was re-opened as a nightclub called the "Moulin Rouge" on 11th December 1957, and after closing in 1974, this use was continued by Mecca Ltd. who re-opened it in January 1975 as "Tiffany's". Stated by the company to be due to poor trading conditions, this closed in March 1981, after which the building was not used and demolished in 1987.

A grill restaurant and the "Natterjack" public house have been erected on the site.

SAVOY/REGENT CINEMA, Preston New Road, Churchtown

The steady, continuous development in the area to the north of Southport of the Churchtown, Hesketh Park and Crossens districts during the 1920's, created a need for entertainment facilities, and it was stated that this would be met in acceptable fashion by the erection of the Savoy Cinema, close to Churchtown railway station on the Southport to Preston line, where it was also easily accessible by the tramcar and bus routes.

The building was designed by Albert Schofield, FRIBA chartered architect of Southport for the proprietors, The Birkdale Picture Palace Co., whose long experience of cinema entertainment dating back to the opening in 1913 of the cinema bearing their name, would, it was considered, enable them to provide all that could be desired as regards up-to-date and varied programmes.

Constructed lengthwise to the main road, the frontage was of multi-coloured bricks and artificial stone, a specially treated preparation which gave the effect of natural stone was a notable feature. The frontage was described as on classic lines, entirely free from all blatant and coarse ornamentation with even special spaces for advertising within stone framed panels. The largest of these was on the taller principal section of the elevation which projected forward of the main building line and included the name of the cinema carved in the stonework above. At either side of this, a short flight of steps led up to an entrance way, beyond which were spacious crush lounges.

Although a stadium-type cinema of only modest size with 750 seats on one main floor, it was reported that the Savoy represented the best traditions of theatre building, incorporating features characteristic of the leading picture houses - atmospheric treatment and rear projection. The former was a decorative style which came into vogue during the 1920's, and so called because it gave to the audience a feeling of being seated in the

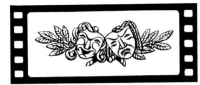

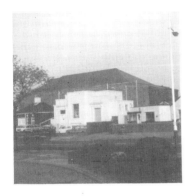

The Savoy, Churchtown had one of the most exotic and unusual auditoria in the country although the frontage was quite traditional. The advert gives details of the grand opening.
Photo: Tony Moss
Drawing: Pat McGowan
Advert: *Southport Visitor*

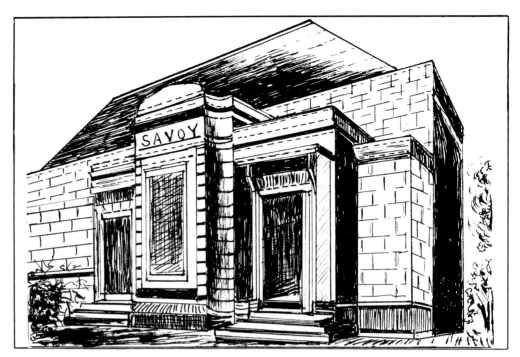

open air beneath a black starry sky amidst various types of scenery. The auditorium of the Savoy was considered a bold adventure in atmospheric treatment with the lower part of the walls representing stone walling with breaks for the entrances and exits. These were adapted to represent entrances to the Italian-style gardens, all grouped with entwining pathways, water-courses, rose gardens and buildings with Romanesque windows. The effectiveness of the scene was enhanced by the fact that the pilot lights of the side gangways were so placed that they appeared as lamp standards within the setting of the ornamental grounds. Designed to obtain perfect harmony, the auditorium ceiling, being elliptical, merged into the walls with a treatment of scenery and sky in one continuous line. Blending with the general scheme, the 30ft proscenium opening, instead of being an isolated unit, was supported on both sides with a Romanesque arcading, being a lead-up from the lower levels. The proscenium pelmet, the stage curtains and the tableaux curtains were of a rich golden colour velvet, enriched with decorative gold applique work of unique design, harmonising with the surroundings. Controlled both from the stage and the operating box, the curtains opened to reveal the cinema screen with purple velvet curtains on either side. A remarkable effect was obtained on all the curtains by the various coloured lighting thrown from the footlights, ceiling batten and spotlights. 'Live' entertainment was provided for, the screen being so arranged that it could be moved right to the back of the stage, allowing space for scenery or stage setting, and reasonable dressing room accommodation was provided.

A feature not in vogue at many cinemas, and the Savoy was the only one in Southport, was "rear projection" which meant that the pictures were shown through the back of the screen. This concentrated the operation of both cine and 'live' entertainment to the stage, the length of which was the picture 'throw' from the projection room at the rear. It was claimed that the system had many advantages such as - no beam along the auditorium, shorter 'throw' no distortion, steadier and clearer pictures. This arrangement also gave the advantage that the operator's room was entirely outside and far away from the auditorium in case of fire, against which great precautions were always necessary in the days of inflammable nitrate film.

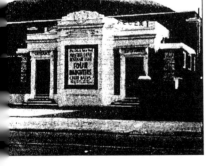

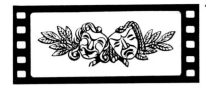

With regard to the seating, those of the first and second class were fitted on a stepped flooring in the rear part of the auditorium, and whilst the general colour scheme was flame colour mohair velvet with mahogany woodwork, the best seats at the back of the hall were covered with rich purple velvet. It was reported that there was ample spacing between the rows, extra wide gangways and that the flooring was covered by a heavy pile carpet.

The auditorium lighting was on the modern, indirect illumination principle, and except for the gangway pilots, not a light in the whole scheme was visible to the audience, thereby facilitating the creation of special lighting effects with colour change.

Described as a paradise for film fans, the Savoy was formally opened by Lieut. Colonel Sir Godfrey Dalrymple-White , MP at 4.00pm on Saturday, 8th December 1928. The cinema was under the management of Mr. W.J. Speakman, who during the previous four years had held a similar position at the Birkdale Picture Palace, with which he was to continue in conjunction with the Savoy. Mr. Speakman was congratulated upon starting his new enterprise with a compliment and an encouragement to British film production by booking as the opening attraction the powerful drama *A Woman Redeemed* featuring Joan Lockton and Brian Aherne. The distinguished patronage also saw an interesting programme of supporting films to piano accompaniment and songs rendered by Miss Nellie Sephton (contralto) and Mr. J.C. Bailey (baritone).

From the following Monday, the cinema was open for evening performances twice nightly at 6.45pm and 8.45pm presenting two programmes weekly changing on Monday and Thursday to which admission prices were 6d, 9d, 1/- and 1/3d.

Early in 1930, Mr. William Walker, the highly esteemed manager of the Coliseum, Southport, during the previous 18 years, took over at the Savoy, also the management of the Birkdale Picture Palace company's other new cinema, the Bedford, Birkdale. The first of many changes made by Mr. Walker at the Savoy was to re-name it the Regent, this was due to the locals having nicknamed it "The Cabbage". Under his management the cinema became one of the most popular in the suburbs of Southport, since in addition to instituting a scheme of modernisation in the style of the thirties, the installation of Western Electric sound system for the opening of the "talkies" was the first outside the town.

Catering once more for all likes and dislikes the management announced that from 3rd May 1930 programmes would consist of "talkies" and "silents" opening with *Does Mother Know Best?* a production of the William Fox studios starring Madge Bellamy and Louise Dresser, and the successful "talkies" on the wonder system - *The Arnaut Brothers*, also several numbers played by the celebrated Gus Arnheim's orchestra. For the latter half of the week the silent feature *Chamber of Horrors* with Frank Stanmore was supported by an excellent "talkie" film *Across the Border* featuring Frank Campeau and Roy Stewart, also the Six Original Brown Brothers in their latest sketch.

Programmes of sound and silent films continued until 10th July when the first All Talking programme featured the film *Flight* starring Jack Holt and Ralph Graves.

Only three years later in May 1933 came the sad news that Mr Walker had died suddenly while viewing a film at the Regent. His death was considered a great loss to the entertainment industry of Southport with which he had been connected since 1906 when he became the general manager of the Empire Theatre, the zoo and the skating rink at the Winter Gardens.

The Regent continued under the same ownership until closing in 1957. Films were then being shown on a wide screen, installed 1956,but although many regular patrons were attending two or three times a week, they were not in sufficient numbers to keep the cinema open. Announcing the closure on 27th May 1957, Mr. J.G. Johnson, general manager, stated that this decision by the Birkdale Picture Palace Co. Ltd. was as a result of excessive entertainment tax from which the recent Budget had given insufficient relief. For the final performance the double feature programme consisted of *So This Is Paris* featuring Tony Curtis, also *Destry* with Audie Murphy.

For many years the building was used as a garage with petrol pumps in the forecourt, until demolition in March 1982 when the present Esso service station was constructed on the site.

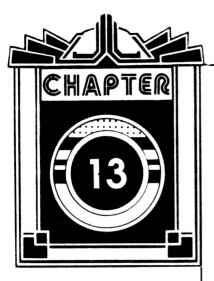

CHAPTER 13

BEDFORD CINEMA, Bedford Road, Birkdale

Opened in 1929 by the Birkdale Picture Palace Co., the Bedford was the last cinema in the Southport area to be opened for the showing of silent films, and the following year provided a more than adequate replacement when the company closed their other cinema in the district, the old Birkdale Picture Palace.

The company, which then also controlled the Savoy, Churchtown, was formed by local businessmen and a Mr Lithgow of Lithgow Nelson, accountants of Lord Street, Southport with Mr Jack Johnson as general manager.

The construction of the auditorium lengthwise to the road provided a 60ft. frontage spanned by a glass verandah about 8ft. deep. The central main entrance was flanked on the left by a sweetshop and on the right by a chemist, and at the extreme right a separate entrance for patrons of the front stalls. Reached by a stairway at the extreme left, the full width of the building at first-floor level was allocated for the projection and rewind rooms, non-sync room and the manager's office.

The main entrance led into a quite wide foyer with entrance doors opposite giving access to the centre and rear of the stadium-type auditorium with a seating capacity of 528. The rear six rows of seats were elevated on a stepped flooring beyond which about twelve rows designated as centre stalls descended on a raked floor to several rows of front stalls. Whereas the company's recently opened Savoy, Churchtown, had the atmospheric decoration of Italian style gardens, the Bedford featured English country scenery with fields and large trees above which the ceiling was treated to represent the sky. Prior to the opening of the Bedford, the company's application to the town council for a 7 day licence was the subject of lengthy meetings during which there was a great amount of arguement for and against Sunday opening. At that time the anomoly existed that whilst all cinemas in the town were permitted to open for one performance at 8.15pm on Sundays in the districts, only the Birkdale Picture Palace and the Queen's, High Park were open on that day. The company proved demand by providing attendance figures over a period for the Picture Palace where they had been larger than on any other evening. After initial refusal, the council reversed their decision shortly after the cinema opened, special programmes on Sundays at 8.15pm were advertised from 11th May 1929.

The opening of the Bedford was not reported in the local press, nor do any records exist to confirm the exact day, and therefore it can only be assumed that this took place on or about the date of the first advertisement, 4th May 1929. Claimed to be the most comfortable cinema in Southport with performances at 3pm, 6.45pm and 8.45pm, the feature film for that day only, Saturday, was *Wild Cat Hetty* featuring Mabel Poulton. 1/-6d and 4d were the prices of admission, reduced to 6d, 4d and 3d for children, and residents in the neighbourhood were soon unanimous in their praise of the type of programmes provided. These were normally double features with three changes weekly.

Early in 1930 the management of the cinema was taken over by the popular and enterprising Mr William Walker of the Coliseum, Southport, in addition to his appointment at the Savoy, Churchtown, where following various improvements and conversion to sound films, Mr Walker similarly equipped the Bedford. Silent films ended on Saturday 1st November 1930 with Harold Lloyd in *Why Worry?* and John Gilbert in *Mask of the Devil*. Equipped with Western Electric sound system on 3rd November the feature film was *King of the Khyber Rifles* featuring Victor McLaglen and Myrna Loy with supporting "shorts" and *British Movietone News*. Admission prices remained the same except for the rear three rows of seats increased to 1/3d.

The cinema survived for nearly thirty years serving a mainly local patronage, who by the 1950's were in decreasing numbers, many making the journey to the town for the first run of the films.

Still under the control of the Birkdale Picture Palace Co. a wide screen was installed in July 1956, but by this time it was little added attraction, and with decreasing attendances for a further 18 months, the Bedford closed on 3rd January 1959 leaving the Embassy, Freshfield, the only surviving cinema in the districts around Southport. The final programme featured the 1958 film of the *Titanic* disaster *A Night to Remember* starring Kenneth More supported by *Gaucho Country*. Matinees having ceased in the early fifties, performances were then continuous in the evenings from 6pm including Sunday, with admission prices at 1/6d, 1/9d and 2/-.

For many years the building was used as a garage, but after closing several years ago, it remains empty up to the present time (1990).

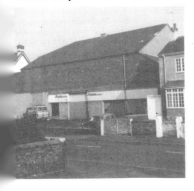

The Bedford, like the Savoy, featured an "atmospheric" auditorium. The walls were decorated to give the impression of being seated in the English countryside, with the ceiling being a simple blue vault to give the impression of the sky.
Photo: Tony Moss

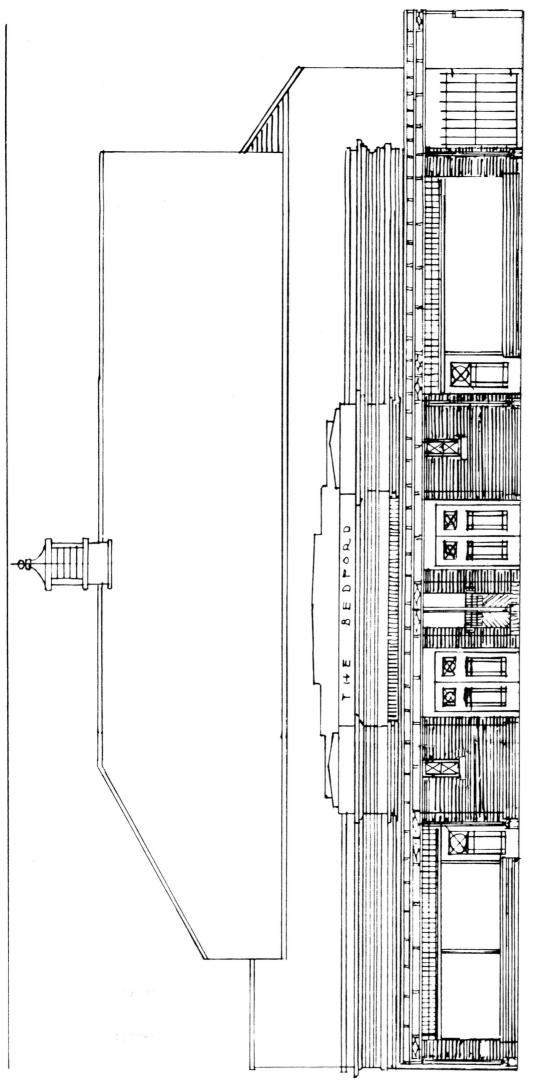

THE BEDFORD

The architect's elevation of the
Bedford shows how detailed the
frontage was, something difficult to
appreciate after the cinema was
turned into a garage.
Elevation: Maxwell Tonge

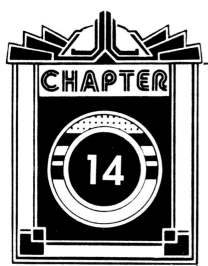

TROCADERO CINEMA, Lord Street, Southport

Originally opened on 29th May 1925 as the Palais de Danse, for four glorious years this building made Southport the dancing mecca of the north-west. The proprietors were Southport Amusements Ltd., and the construction was to the plans of Southport architect George Tonge, who went on to make his mark in Art Deco buildings that typified the 1930's and was one of a set of classical edifices in Portland stone built around London Square in harmony with the town's war memorial of 1923 in front of the building.

The long frontage, 135ft across was parallel to the length of the building, and had a central main entrance way flanked on either side by shops. The entrance was a most imposing feature divided into three separate ways between four pairs of tall columns which supported an entablature high above the portico. This was at the head of several steps with a flooring of large black and white marble squares, and had three pairs of doors to a wide foyer with large booking office in dark oak, panelled walls and Japanese-style lanterns suspended from the ceiling. This was the first indication of the decorative style, the dominant note being Japanese and it was stated that the glamour of the Far East was spread over the scenes of gaiety, which were characteristic of the beautiful building.

At that time the largest dance hall in the north-west, the ballroom was magnificent with a 10,000 square foot parquet floor laid on 1,000 springs and accommodated 1,500 dancers. Numerous Japanese lanterns of various shapes and sizes illuminated the ballroom, suspended from the curved ceiling, and around the edge at a height of 8ft was a balcony used as a cafe with tables and chairs between the columns from which spectators could watch the dancers and be served by waitresses with refreshments, including afternoon tea at 1s 6d. The modern American soda fountains dispensed ice-cream in a great variety of flavours from the Palais own ice-cream factory which supplied some of the town's cinemas. The first resident band was that of Billy Cotton and the Palais was his first step to fame. International cabaret was presented almost every week and included many famous names, of these now the best remembered is Fred Astaire.

The departure of Billy Cotton and his band to the newly opened Rialto, Liverpool in October 1927 began the decline of the Palais, although its premature closure in 1929 was as a result of a scandal, a sensational court case following a waitress's allegations regarding the conduct of persons in rooms allocated for private dancing lessons! Soon after this, in 1929 the building was closed for conversion into a 'talkie' cinema.

Having an imposing facade with columned main entrance, according with the architectural style of nearby edifices, and in addition, a spacious auditorium, the Palais de Danse was considered eminently suitable to satisfy all the requirements of a super-cinema. It was nevertheless realised that the conversion would be a difficult operation requiring careful consideration, but fortunately the right man for the task was at hand, Mr. George E. Tonge, FRIBA, the architect of the original building, and to him was entrusted the drawing up of plans for the entire scheme. On completion it was stated that the original lines of the building had been admirably preserved, the appearance of the interior having an agreeable familiarity combined with a fresh modern treatment.

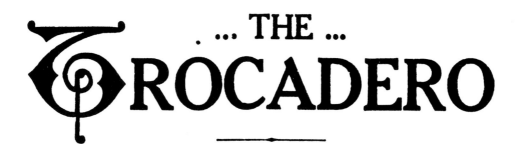

... THE ...

TROCADERO

SOUTHPORT'S NEW CINEMA DE LUXE.

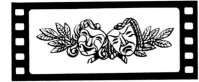

From the foyer, glass panelled doors opposite the main entrance gave access to a long corridor with curtained entrances to the left-hand side of the auditorium, where it was stated, the cinema ideal of an unobstructed view of the screen from every part of the house was achieved. The seating in the front part was on a gradual slope, beyond which, separated by a crossover gangway, eighteen rows were fitted on a stepped flooring up to the level of the side balconies at the rear. The seating capacity on the main floor was 1,280, later increased to 1,357 with seats on the balconies; all were upholstered in blue plush and the floor covered by a rich, amber-toned carpet, and wide gangways extended around the entire hall with ample exits at points of easy access.

A large stage with orchestra pit in front, also commodious dressing room accommodation provided for the possibility of variety acts being included in the performances. The straight-topped proscenium of approximately 40ft width was described as effectively designed with tastefully elegant drapes and artistic lighting effects, and the flanking walls included an exit way, and above, a full length ornamental grille was surmounted by a large letter 'T' for Trocadero, as the cinema was to be named. The decorations and appointments excellently conformed to the modern ideal with charming colour schemes of the ceiling and the walls whilst the principal illumination of the hall was from lamps within multi-coloured glass shaded fittings, fitted flush with the curved ceiling.

At the rear of the hall was constructed the new projection suite with rewind and tonal control rooms, claimed to be one of the finest in the country equipped with the latest machines connected to the new Western Electric sound system.

TROCADERO

Tel. 3674.   SOUTHPORT'S PREMIER CINEMA.   Tel. 3674.

Week Commencing MONDAY NEXT, OCTOBER 28th, 1929, at 2-45. 6-40 and 8-50.

FIRST SHOWING IN SOUTHPORT.

ALL TALKING, SINGING, DANCING, DRAMATIC SENSATION.

THE BROADWAY MELODY

WITH

CHARLES KING, ANITA PAGE, BESSIE LOVE.

The Film that has smashed every record in Theatre History wherever shown.
THE MIRACLE OF THE TALKING SCREEN.

GRAND OPENING PERFORMANCE, Monday Next, Oct. 28th, at 2-30 p.m.
Under the Distinguished Patronage of HIS WORSHIP THE MAYOR & MAYORESS.
Special Prices this Performance only: Stalls, 1/-; Royal Stalls, 2/-.

PRICES OF ADMISSION:
Evenings 6d., 1/-, 1/6, 2/- limited number.   6d. Bargain Matinees that "TALK." 600 Seats at 6d. (also 1/- & 1/6).
Advance Booking Office Open Daily from 10 a.m. to 8 p.m.

As a magnificent ballroom the Trocadero only lasted for four years. The opening advert describes the Trocadero as Southport's premier cinema.
Advert: *Southport Visitor*

Described as the last word in cinema construction and styled as Southport's Cinema-de-Luxe, the Trocadero was opened by the former proprietors, Southport Amusements Ltd, under the management of Mr. Will Hughes, whose popularity at the Palladium was founded on a sound judgement of the public taste and an enterprising ability to gratify it. The Grand Opening of the town's then largest cinema took place at 2.30pm on Monday 28th October 1929, when the opening ceremony was performed by the Mayor in the presence of an audience which included members of the Town Council, magistracy and other leading townspeople. The feature film was the first showing in Southport of the All Talking, Singing and Dancing sensation, MGM's *The Broadway Melody* featuring Charles King, Anita Page and Bessie Love. The film had smashed every record in cinema history wherever shown and advance booking was advised, for which the box office was to be open from 10am to 8pm. For the special opening matinee admission was at 1/- and 2/- thereafter at 6d, 1/- , 1/6d and 2/- to the 6.40pm and 8.50pm evening performances, whilst 600 seats at 6d were available to the bargain matinees at 2.45pm.

Although opening as a 'talkie' cinema with *The Broadway Melody* running for two weeks followed by *The Trial of Mary Dugan* MGM's first all-dialogue film featuring Norma Shearer for one week commencing 11th November, there followed a short season of silent films accompanied by the Grand Symphony Orchestra led by T.W. Kottaun. The 'talkies'

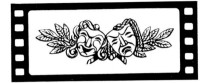

returned on 6th January 1930 with Ruth Chatterton in *Madame X* also supporting programme including *British Movietone News*. On 7th July 1930 the public inauguration of the Compton wonder organ was announced, stated to be a masterpiece of modern ingenuity and technical skill. It was played by Herbert A. Dowson formerly organist at the Tivoli, Strand, London. Organ interludes continued during the '30's, for a time in 1937 by Dixon Burrell advertised as "The Boy Wonder" and in November 1938, Herbert Dowson became the organist at the new Grand Cinema, Lord Street.

Following periods of only occasional use during the '40's, and out of use in the '50's, the organ at the Trocadero was removed in 1961, with the general clearing out of the furniture and fittings after the closure of the cinema in October 1960. Surprisingly, it was nearly 25 years later when the location of the instrument was traced by the Cinema Organ Society, who discovered that it was erected in the West Gallery of Parkend Church in the Forest of Dean.

The Trocadero and the company's other cinema on Lord Street, the Forum, were operated by Associated Southport Cinemas as lessees from 1938 until the mid-40's, after which they were under the control of the proprietors, Grand Cinema (Southport) Ltd.

Due to the increased competition from the major circuits from 1938, when in addition to Gaumont British, ABC were also represented in the town with the opening of the Regal, the availability of first-run films to the Trocadero was considerably reduced, and gradually losing its status as a first-run cinema, by the '50's it was mainly restricted to later runs and 'B' pictures. The position did not improve until 1954, although even then, as it transpired, only for a limited time. The Trocadero was then one of the many independent cinemas throughout the country, and the first in Southport to be equipped for CinemaScope with four-track magnetic stereophonic sound. This new projection system was pioneered and developed by Twentieth Century Fox, who guaranteed first run of their releases in this format, to all exhibitors who installed the complete equipment. The complete package included a special curved wide screen with aspect ratio of 2.55 to 1, the width being over 2 1/2 times that of the height. Behind this, a line of speakers gave directional sound according to the position of its source on the screen and the realism was further enhanced by additional speakers mounted on the auditorium walls for special effects.

The Trocadero was designed by George E. Tonge who had designed the original building to harmonise with the war memorial.
Photo: W.E. Marsden

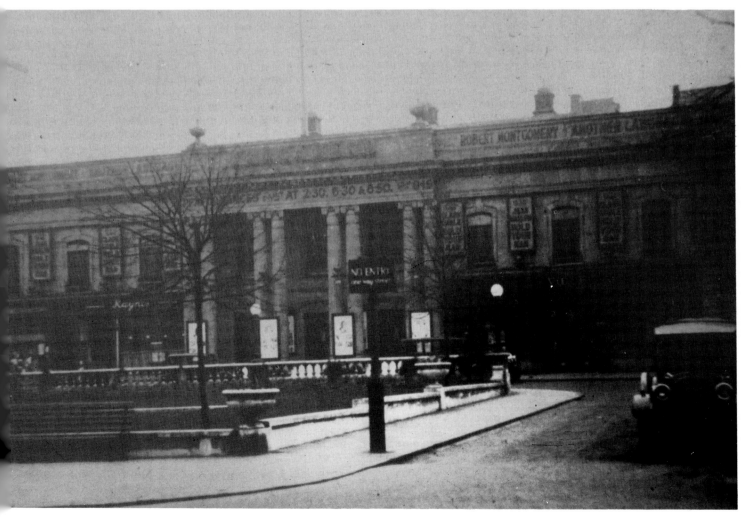

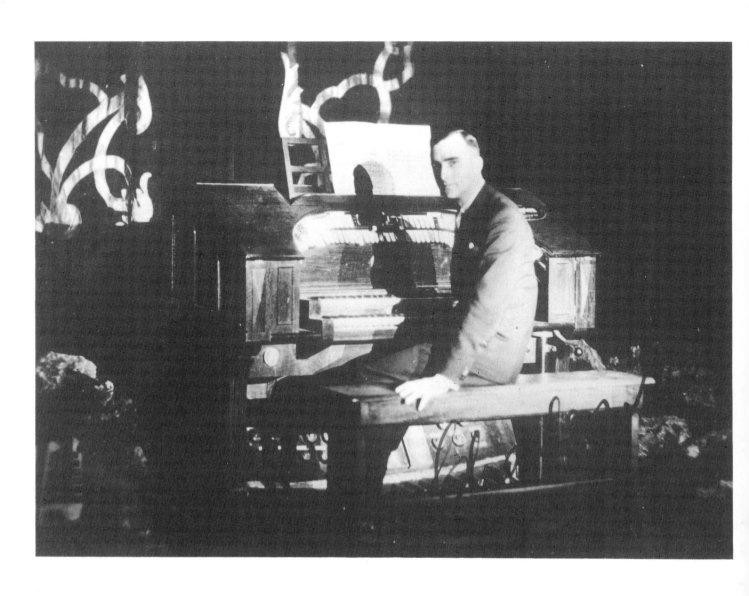

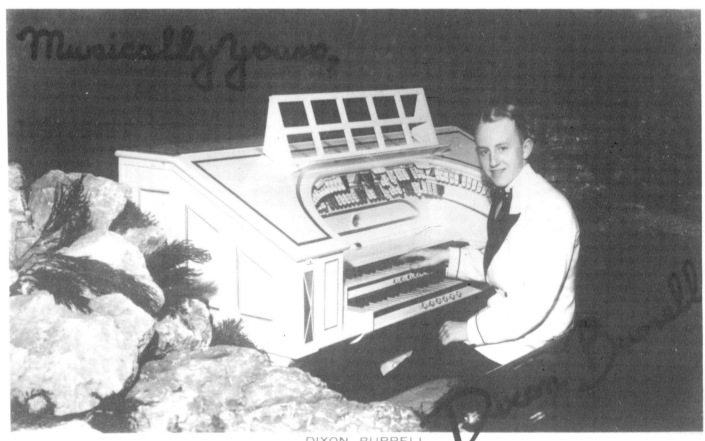

DIXON BURRELL
AT THE ORGAN OF THE TROCADERO CINEMA SOUTHPORT

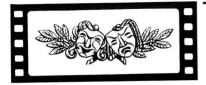

The Compton organ was originally played by Herbert Dowson, the public inauguration taking place on 7th July 1930. In 1937 it was played for a while by Dixon Burrell, "The Boy Wonder", shown in the lower photo. The upper photo shows C. Massey.
Photos: John Sharp

The elevation of the screen end of the auditorium gives an idea of the decorative scheme.
Elevation: Metropolitan Borough of Sefton

The Trocadero announced on 12th April 1954 - "The silver screen moves into the Golden Age of CinemaScope" with the first CinemaScope film, *The Robe*, featuring Richard Burton and Jean Simmons, preceded by a special documentary explaining the principles of the new projection system, at three performances daily, 2.30, 5.25 and 8.05pm.

Although this proved a considerable boost to attendances at the Trocadero, other cinemas in the town soon opened with CinemaScope, although minus stereophonic sound, but this too was included six months later at the company's leading cinema, the Grand, which took over first run of the Fox releases. The Trocadero then reverted back to its former film booking policy, and after a further six years with declining admissions, near the end of September 1960, the company announced imminent closure, having sold the building and site for re-development as an extension to Woolworth's stores through to Lord Street.

The Trocadero closed on 1st October 1960 with a continuous performance from 2.15pm of a double feature programme - *The Planter's Wife* starring Claudette Colbert and Jack Hawkins, also *Never Say Goodbye* featuring Rock Hudson.

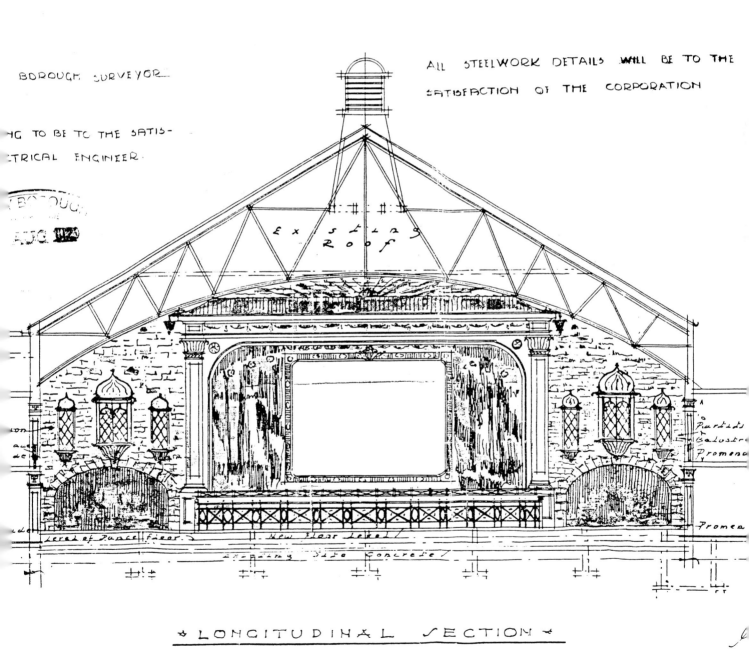

LONGITUDINAL SECTION

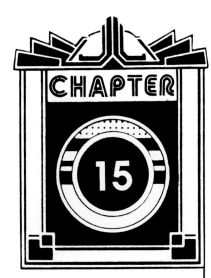

CHAPTER

15

EMBASSY CINEMA, Green Lane, Freshfield

The local press of 9th April 1932 announced that the district possessed a house of distinction of the cinema world in the Embassy, described as a handsomely appointed picture house, and an excellent conversion from its former use as the Embassy Hall skating rink, erected in 1928.

Constructed lengthwise to the road, the ground floor of the frontage was allocated for several shops and, at the extreme left, a garage with petrol pumps in the forecourt, whilst at the extreme right, the main entrance to the cinema was surmounted by a small canopy with the name EMBASSY on the front against a background of white opaque glass. The upper part of the frontage was constructed of brick relieved by white plaster-covered areas around the six large windows, and in the centre, a panel indicated the year of erection - 1928.

Internally the former skating rink on the first floor was converted into the stalls area of the cinema, and a shallow balcony provided seating accommodation for 714. The main entrance gave access to the rear of the stalls and balcony whilst for the front of the stalls a separate entrance on the opposite side of the building was provided. Beyond the main entrance, staircases with artistic balustrades led up to the first floor, where at either side was a comfortable lounge furnished with mahogany armchairs. Via a short flight of stairs these led to the rear of the balcony at either side, where the seats were enclosed by a highly polished wood panelled screen. These were also erected behind the rear row of stalls seats. Due to the squarish shape of the hall the seats were fitted in three sections across, with fewer than normal number of rows from front to rear. This particularly affected the arrangement in the balcony where the space in the centre was restricted by the projection room, and sufficient for only a few rows of seats. Most of these were at either side, which was fortunate, since patrons walking to their seats in the centre obstructed the light beam from the low projection ports. All tip-up seats were provided, rexine-covered in the front stalls, Lister's "Dreadnought" velvet seats at the rear and more elaborate seats of the same material in the balcony, all on a floor covered by Wilton carpet.

The auditorium featured a 40ft wide proscenium, and illuminated scenic panels, one a Canadian, the other an Eastern scene at either side, also a stage to provide for the possibility of 'live' entertainment. The walls were adorned by decorative panels and the decorations described as tasteful and striking, avoiding the bizarre treatment to be found in some cinemas. Including the decorative and stage lighting there were 400 lighting points, the installation of which was carried out by the engineer of the proprietor, Wigan Entertainments Ltd, but as at all cinemas of that time, secondary lighting was by gas.

A cinematograph and a dancing licence was applied for on behalf of Councillor F. Worswick, and under the management of Mr. Bernard Worswick, advertised as "The House of Distinction" the Embassy opened on Wednesday, 6th April 1932 with performances at 6.15pm and 8.45pm. Equipped with Western Electric sound system there was a double feature comprised *Toast of the Legion* with Walter Pidgeon and Bernice Claire, also *Little Caesar* featuring Edward G. Robinson. The prices of admission were 7d and 1/- in the stalls, and 1/6d in the balcony, children at half price and seats were bookable in advance. For the latter half of the week the programme was changed to *Devotion* starring Ann Harding, with the supporting feature *The Sundown Trail* one performance nightly at 7.30pm, which was to be the normal time except for Wednesday and Saturday.

Although as in the case of Southport's other suburban cinemas, films were screened at dates considerably later than at those in the town, the Embassy nevertheless remained open until 1962, when for three years it had been the only cinema in the districts around Southport. Apparently no records exist to indicate the actual date of closure, and the task of tracing this has been made virtually impossible since, with the exception of the opening, the cinema had no advertisements in the local press, suggesting an almost entirely local patronage.

For a short time the Embassy reverted to its original purpose as an ice rink, then being used as a carpet warehouse until 1976 and a furniture store until the mid-eighties. This was followed by a period of closure for about 12 months, when it was converted for the opening in 1986 as the Embassy Snooker Centre.

With the exception that a supermarket has replaced the garage at the left hand side, the frontage still includes a short row of shops up to the main entrance of the snooker hall and has changed little from its early days.

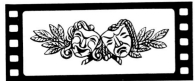

The Embassy was originally an ice rink and after closure as a cinema, reverted to its original use before becoming a carpet warehouse. After a period as a furniture store it has become a snooker hall. The frontage remains relatively unchanged.
Photo: Mrs Yorke, Formby Society

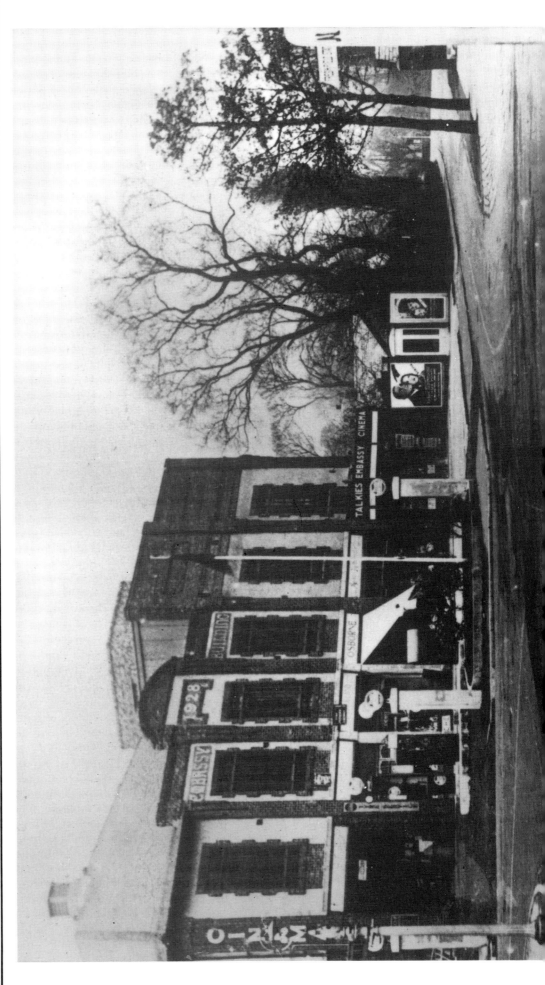

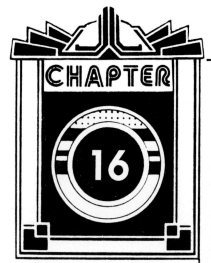

CHAPTER 16

The building contractors made a scale model of the Floral Hall which was displayed to the public, creating a great deal of interest.
Photo: Metropolitan Borough of Sefton

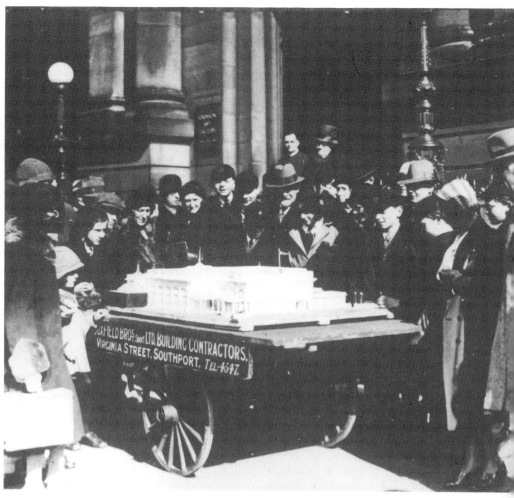

THE FLORAL HALL, Promenade, Southport

To the many attractions of which Southport could boast in 1932 was added the new Floral Hall, constructed on the north side of the pier in the midst of the sunken rose gardens, which were brought into the scheme to make the enterprise of the corporation a wonderfully pleasing and charming centre of attraction, described as a rendezvous of entertainment and pleasure unrivalled throughout the country. To the plans of Southport architects, Messrs Archer & Gooch, F/LRIBA, the flat-roofed building was stated to have been designed on classic lines with a long, low plaster-faced frontage in white, spaced along which were pairs of columns extending up to the coping. The ultra modern note of the thirties was in evidence due to the large beautifully designed windows, which together with the unusual system of external lighting by quaint Japanese-style lanterns, and many hued umbrellas gave a charming atmosphere of gaiety. The main entrance to the hall originally faced the lake with two wide stairways leading down from the promenade on either side of the building providing a ready means of access for all pedestrians, whilst cars and other vehicles were given ample parking space.

Described as impressive by its spaciousness, the large square-shaped auditorium, seated 1,600 with magnificent stage and attractive proscenium in the art deco style of the thirties with plain, plaster-faced surfaces relieved by modest designs in contrasting darker colour. The stage, 48 ft. in width and 26 ft. deep with ample dressing and storage accommodation, provided facilities for all types of performances. The proscenium was adorned by a pelmet of deep red with a gold border and matching drapes which opened to reveal the gold-coloured stage curtain with deep festooned pelmet. The stage was illuminated by overhead magazine battens taking the place of the usual footlights, this arrangement allowed a completely clear stage, the lighting of which was sub-divided into white, red, blue or green, varied or collectively by hand-operated dimmers. The proscenium lighting and stage floods were from a number of spotlighting lanterns fixed in the ceiling and at the front and rear of the central dome.

In the front portion of the hall an area of approximately 900 square yards was laid with a suitable sprung floor, with special lighting effects above for the purpose of dancing.

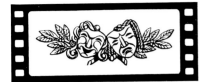

The Floral Hall no longer has the imposing look displayed here since the adjacent Southport Theatre has been built.
Photo: Metropolitan Borough of Sefton

The principal lighting of the auditorium was by 13 artistic, hexagonal-shaped lanterns panelled with opalescent amber-coloured glass and curved corners in green, of which the light metal framework of the fittings and suspension tubes in emerald green were stated to harmonize day and night with the decor.

The considerable width of the hall, approximately 90 ft. allowed space at the front right-hand side for a cafe, capable of meeting the anticipated heavy demand, whilst on either side of the hall, glass-panelled doors with a sun-ray design led onto corridors from which there was access to the gardens.

The Floral Hall was not only planned for 'live' entertainment, concerts and dancing, but was also adaptable for wrestling, and public meetings were also held there. However, the distinction of giving the first performance for the Grand Opening on Whit Monday, 16 May 1932 went to the Southport Orpheus Operatic Society's production of the Gilbert & Sullivan opera *The Gondoliers* which delighted the distinguished audience including the Lord Mayor & Lady Mayoress, Councillor and Mrs. W.H. Bellis, members of the Town Council and corporation officials.

In more recent years a new main entrance with canopy was constructed at the left-hand side of the frontage, but this was re-styled as the entrance to the Lounge Bar in 1972 due to the creation of an entertainment complex including the Southport Theatre. Since that time there has been an additional entrance to the right-hand side of the Floral Hall from the new foyer of the theatre, which is in a central position between the two auditoria, and that of the Floral Hall has a licensed bar in the area of the former cafe.

The Floral Hall continues to present such varied entertainment as concerts, old time Music Hall, Band shows, musical groups, talent contests, dancing and wrestling, forming a worthy contrast to the big name variety shows at the adjacent Southport Theatre.

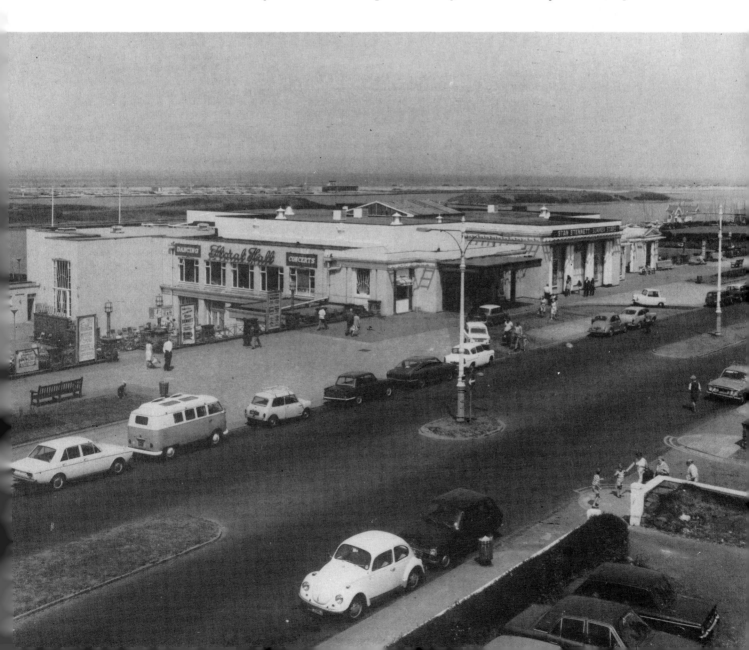

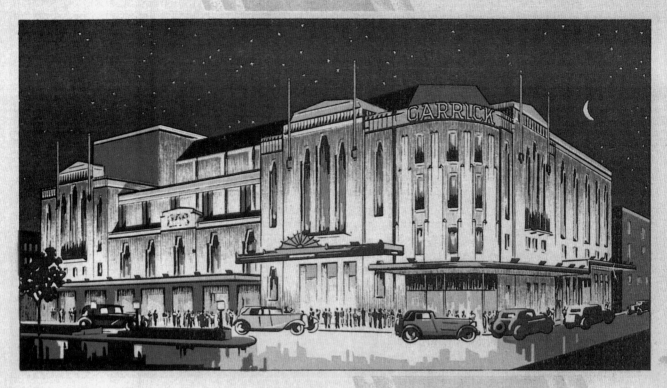

The most beautiful Theatre in Europe presenting the finest Plays, Revues & Variety programmes.

The Book of the
Garrick
THEATRE
SOUTHPORT

The above picture is from a souvenir booklet given to patrons. The others on these pages are from the opening brochure.
Pictures: Mike Yelland (above) and Metropolitan Borough of Sefton

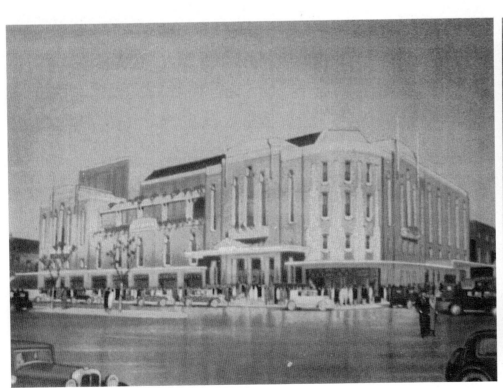

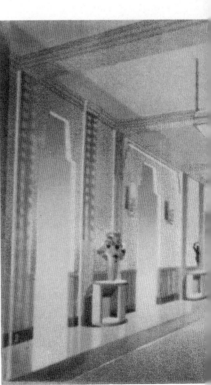

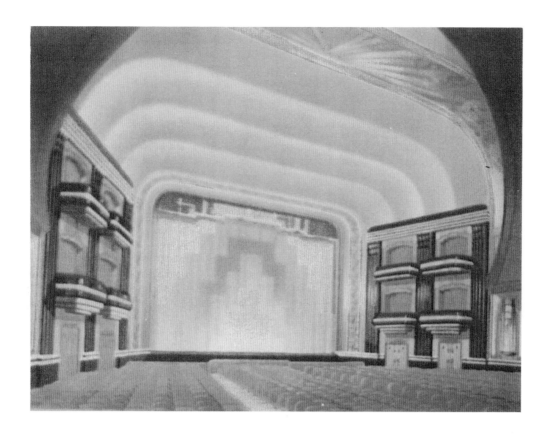

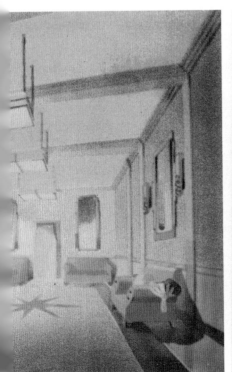

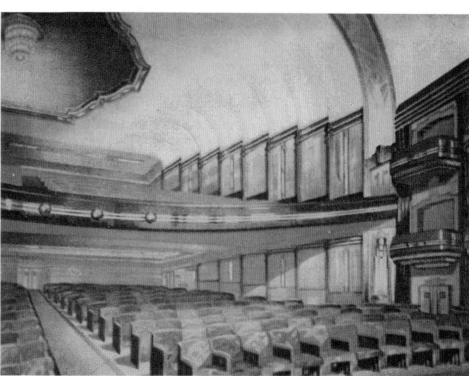

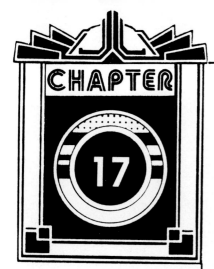

CHAPTER 17

GARRICK THEATRE/ESSOLDO. Lord Street, Southport.

The opening of the Garrick Theatre was considered a notable event ranking high in the annals of Southport, restoring the resort to its former place as one of the most enterprising centres of entertainment in the North. Erected at a cost of £120,000 on the site of the Opera House, destroyed by fire in December 1929, the Garrick was the most modern theatre in the country vying in artistic splendour with the best in London and the Continental capitals.

Described as a monument to the owner, Mr. George Rose, and reflecting great credit on the well-known local architect, Mr. George E. Tonge, the building constituted from a structural point of view a magnificent addition to the architectural elegance of the town and the claim that Lord Street was one of the finest thoroughfares in the country. The fact that the Opera House was so soon replaced by the Garrick Theatre was due to the enterprise of George Rose and son, Harry, London and Manchester businessmen who formed the Southport Theatre Co. acquiring the site of the former theatre. In the early thirties when particularly the provincial theatres were fighting a losing battle against the challenge of the talking cinema, it required considerable courage to initiate such an enterprise, but this was done in the only possible way, by erecting a theatre surpassing the magnificence of the super cinema. The architect, Mr. George E. Tonge, LRIBA, was stated to have carried out a finely conceived design in the Italian Renaissance style adding lustre to his reputation as the author of brilliant schemes for modern entertainment houses.

Prominently situated on an island site at the junction of Lord Street and Kingsway, frontages to both linked by a curved corner were of rustic brick relieved by stone. At the extreme right of the Lord Street frontage, the main entrance, divided into three separate ways by square columns was surmounted by an individual ornamented canopy set at a higher level than that of the principal length extending along the frontages in which were incorporated several shops. Above first floor level the Lord Street elevation was fronted by an open air colonnade and ornamental gardens for use by patrons during the summer months.

The artists sketches of the waiting areas of the Garrick show how elegant the building was. It was described as a monument to the owner, the Garrick must surely have been George Tonge's best design. Drawings: *Southport Star*

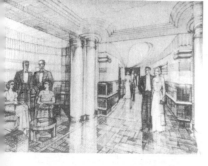

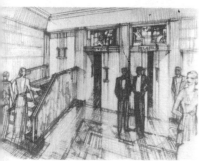

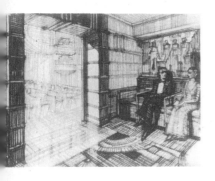

The main entrance led into the spacious foyer in which the domed ceiling and niches containing statuary were notable features. Decoration was in the Egyptian style with walls and ceiling of black glass striped with silver. This area gave access on the left to the rear stalls whilst a broad, thickly carpeted staircase led up to the circle lounge and entrances.

Including the spacious balcony and boxes the auditorium had a seating capacity of 1,600, and upon entering the eye was immediately drawn to the magnificent 50ft. wide proscenium, given prominence set between the long, splayed flanking walls in which on either side were four boxes on two levels above the two front stalls exits. Further enhancing the appearance of the proscenium, the ceiling followed its contours with concealed lighting in troughs of increasing width along the splayed walls. This area of the ceiling was bordered by a broad band of plasterwork in red and gold, whilst at ground floor level an attractive feature was provided by recesses with elegant light fittings.

The stage, one of the largest in the provinces, designed to accommodate the big productions was equipped with the latest devices in connection with lighting, scenery shifting mechanism, fireproof curtain etc.

On completion of the building, comment was made on the rapid construction, for although the foundation stone was not laid until 25th February 1932, the theatre was ready for opening in less than ten months on 19th December. This was the date on which Mr. Rose had insisted, being the date of his wedding anniversary, having built the theatre for his wife, who had regularly attended the Opera House.

Amid scenes of great enthusiasm the Garrick Theatre was opened on 19th December 1932, and from the moment when the floodlights were switched on, illuminating the facade, surmounted with flags of many nations, the excitement of the crowd reached a climax when a fanfare of trumpets heralded the raising of the curtain at 7pm when the formal opening was performed by the famous actor Sir John Martin Harvey. Presiding over the opening ceremony, the Mayor of Southport, Councillor G.E. Hardman was supported by the actor, George and Harry Rose and many town councillors. Following many speeches from the stage the curtain rose at 8pm on the new mystery drama *Firebird* from the London Playhouse, with Miss Gladys Cooper and the full London company. The prices of admission reflected the high standard of entertainment offered at this and subsequent performances, being fixed at 4/6 and 5/6 in the circle, 5/- and 6/- in the stalls whilst the boxes were at £2.

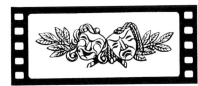

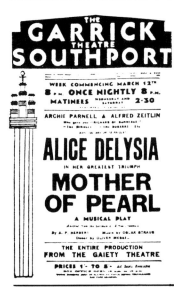

During the following 25 years the Garrick presented every type of 'live' entertainment - operas, musical comedies, drama, summer shows and Christmas pantomimes, but in January 1957, the proprietor, Victor Sheridan, announced the sale of the theatre to the Newcastle-based Essoldo cinema circuit. His reason was that being the country's third largest entertainment circuit, they would be in a more favourable position to continue the presentation of big stage productions.

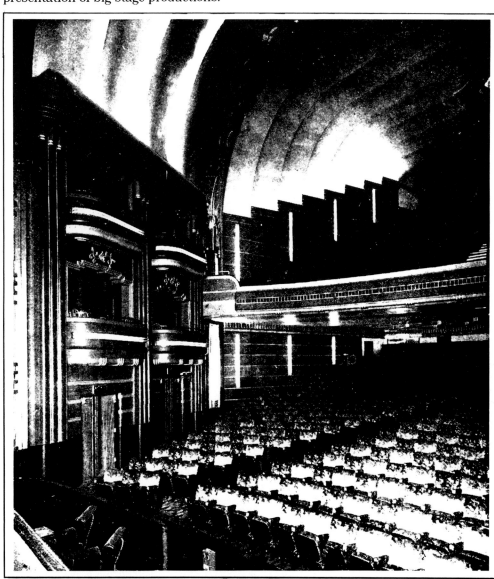

The auditorium (right) plus the staff (below) comprising usherettes, call boys and orchestra give an idea of the opulance the Garrick exuded. Photos: Michael Yelland

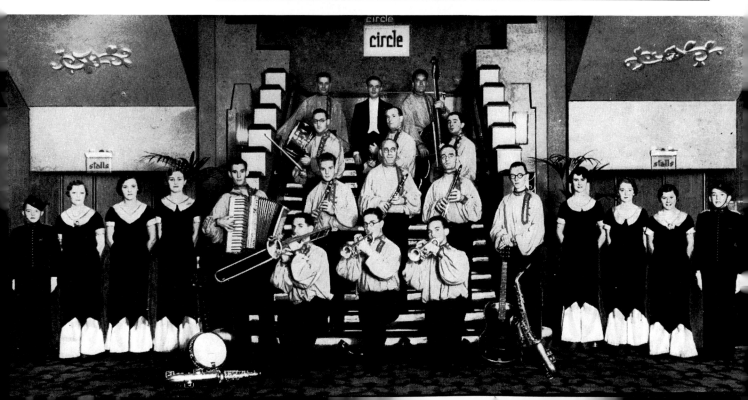

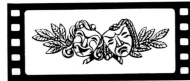

Like so many cinemas, the Garrick was renamed. It became the Essoldo in the late 1950s. In March 1971 the Palace was renamed the Essoldo, a name it kept for just over a year until it was taken over by Classic Cinemas, under whose control it was again known as the Palace until opened as Classic 1 & 2 on 12th May 1974.
Advert: *Southport Journal*, Wednesay 10th July 1963

Pages 93, 94 and 95 show the imposing exterior of the Garrick. The photo opposite was taken shortly before opening. Those on pages 94 and 95 show the Garrick under Ladbroke's control as a "Lucky 7" bingo club.
Photos: Michael Yelland

The Garrick remained relatively the same to look at after bingo took over as these two photos below show. Even today, as the Top Rank Club, the building is still the landmark it was the day it opened as the Garrick.
Photos: C. Cramp (below) and Mike Taylor (bottom)

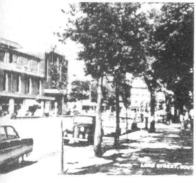

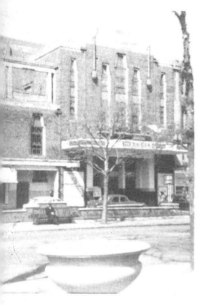

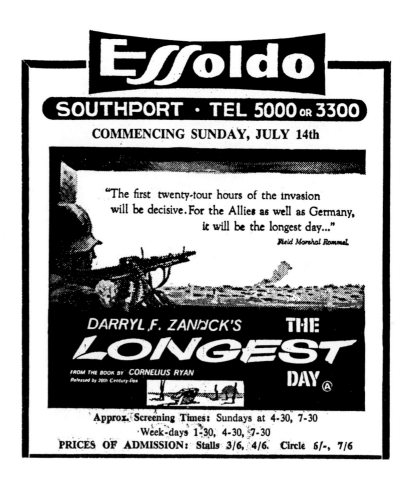

Essoldo stated their intention to re-open the Garrick as a cinema, but revert back to live entertainment with a first class summer show and a pantomime at Christmas. Stage shows were temporarily ended on 19th January 1957 with the pantomime *Robin Hood* on Ice. After the final curtain an army of electrical engineers and technicians commenced the work of equipping the Garrick as a cinema, working non-stop until Monday morning so that all would be completed for the doors opening at 1.30pm. The theatre's former spotlight box was converted into a projection room and equipped by G.B. Kalee Ltd. with two G.B. Kalee 20 projectors, "president' arcs and 30 watt amplifier. On the stage, a "Perlux' the latest in British cinema screens was mounted on a 46ft. by 22ft. tubular frame and tilted back 7 degrees to counteract the projection rake of 24 degrees. Movable black masking altered the picture size for all formats from normal and wide screen to a CinemaScope size of 37ft. by 17ft.

With seating reduced to 1,500, all the same standard of comfort and prices ranging from 1/6d to 3/9d, the Garrick opened as a cinema on 21st January 1957 with a continuous performance from 2pm of the CinemaScope film *Love Me Tender* starring Elvis Presley also *Miracle on 34th Street* with Maureen O'Hara.

As a cinema, the Garrick was never very successful, due to strong competition from the ABC, Odeon and other leading cinemas, showing first run films. By the end of the fifties, the name Garrick was dispensed with in favour of Essoldo in accordance with company policy. With attendances for films in decline, the company allocated many dates for stage shows, but in May 1962, the lack of support for these too was the subject of a front page article in the local press following a comment from manager Vernon Hunter. During 1963 bingo sessions were introduced on Sundays and Fridays, and in November of that year, by which time the club membership had grown to 4,000, the change to full-time bingo was announced, Those who wished to remember the Essoldo as a cinema were advised that they had five days during the week ending 16th November to see *Tom Jones* featuring Albert Finney, of which there were three performances daily at 2.35pm, 5.20pm and 8.05pm.

With a change of name to the Lucky Seven bingo was continued in the seventies by Ladbrokes Ltd. who expended a considerable sum on refurbishment and in 1984 the hall became a Top Rank bingo club.

A night-time study of the floodlit GARRICK

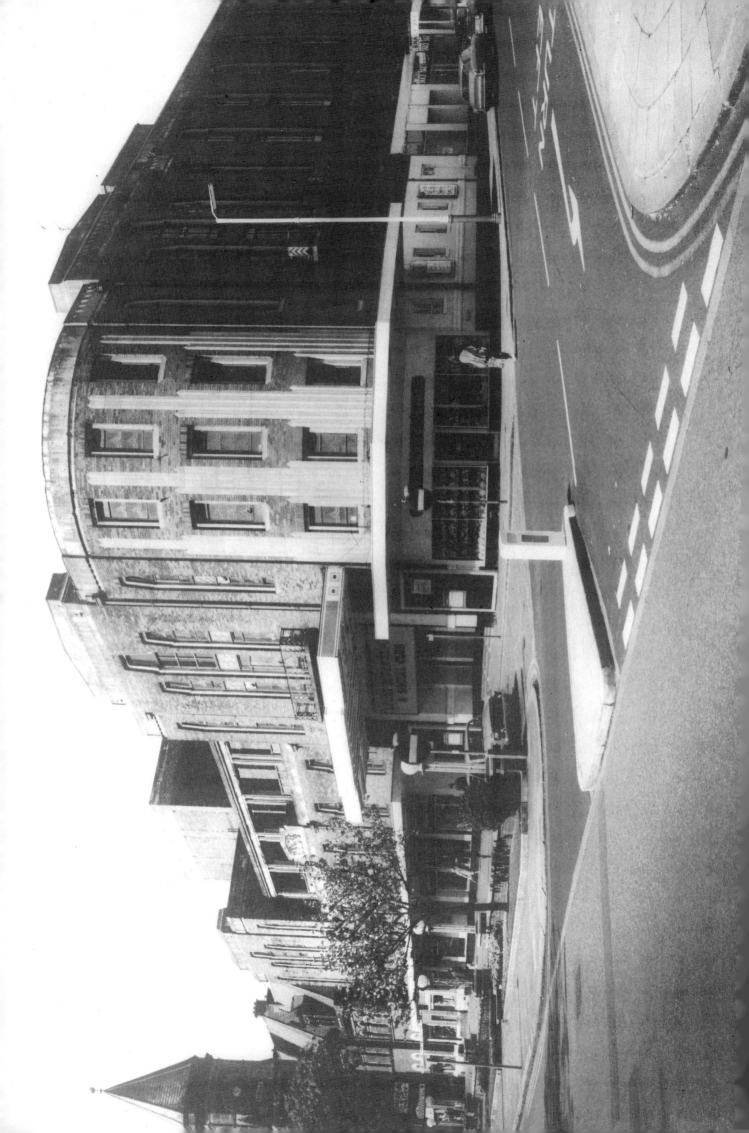

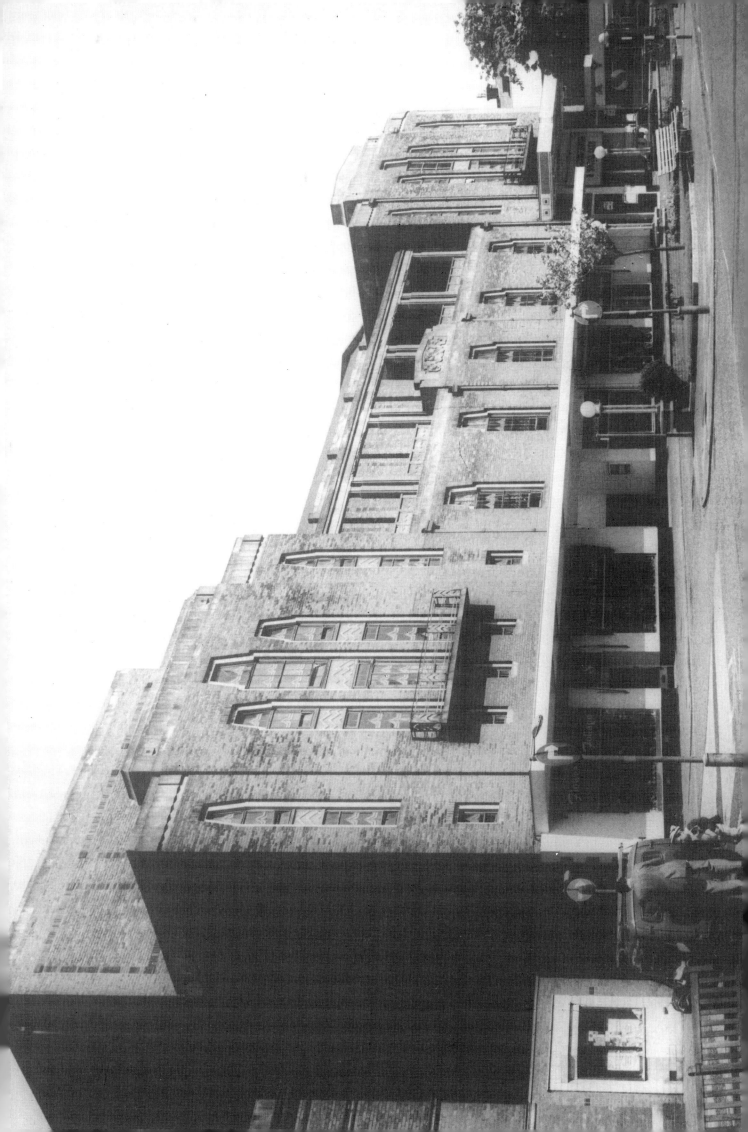

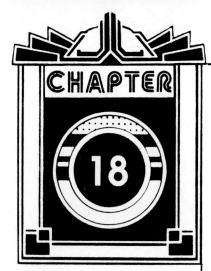

LITTLE THEATRE, Hoghton Street, Southport

Although hidden unobtrusively away at the rear of Victoria House, the Little Theatre has for over 50 years been among the town's most important venues for theatregoers as the home of the Southport Dramatic Club.

Dating back to 1913 the club had its beginning at the flourishing St. Andrews School in Part Street where a number of the older girls formed their own dramatic society under the leadership of Miss Elsie Leivesley, who may be termed the founder of the S.D.C. Before the First World War the St. Andrews Old Girls Dramatic Society produced Tennyson's *Princess Ida* in the school hall, which later proved to be too small resulting in a move to the Temperance Institute. After the war, the society's progress was maintained, enabling them to hire the Palladium, and in 1919 for the first time, men took part in the society's activities. Soon afterwards the name was changed, the Southport Dramatic Club being officially founded in 1920.During the 1920s the club's annual production was presented for one week each winter at the Opera House until the disastrous fire in December 1929. 1931 saw the club at the much smaller Pier Pavilion Theatre, where, for the first time more than one play was produced during the rather short time at this location. The S.D.C. then only two years later moved to the new Garrick Theatre erected on the site of the Opera House, presenting two plays during the winter, before taking steps to acquiring a permanent home in 1934. The members rented two rooms over a garage in Mornington Road, in which they built a stage, and in astonishingly cramped conditions, succeeded in producing a considerable number of plays to capacity audiences of 75!

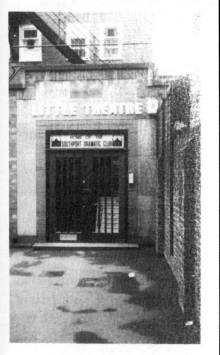

Although only a small entrance, the auditorium is relatively large. The Little Theatre remains a popular venue for Southport's theatregoers. Photos: Chris Clegg (above) and Michael Yelland (opposite)

When Victoria House was erected by the Liverpool Victoria Friendly Society, club officials began prolonged negotiations resulting in the building of a full sized theatre at the rear of these premises. The architect of the theatre was Albert Schofield, FRIBA. and on 24th October 1936 the ceremony of laying the foundation stone was performed by the club's president, Sir Barry Jackson, M.A. Funded and equipped by money provided by the 4I founder members, the Little Theatre opened on 2nd October 1937 with the S.D.C's production of *Dear Brutus* by J.M. Barrie. at 8pm with admission at 1/6d,, 2/6d and 3/6d.

From Hoghton Street the only indications of the theatre are the advertising frames flanking the entrance way on the right-hand side of Victoria House giving access to a spacious courtyard on which the front entrance of the theatre is directly opposite at the far end. Extending to the left from the entrance doors, the foyer accommodated the booking office and a telephone kiosk, the former originally at the foot of the wide segmental staircase on the left-hand side, which curves up to and terminates in the crush hall leading into a large foyer, both giving direct access to the rear of the auditorium. The original seating capacity was 430 with particular attention to providing an uninterrupted view of the stage, the seats, in two blocks with centre and side gangways being generously spaced on a well-raked floor. The decorative treatment of the side walls created the illusion of added length, being in broad horizontal bands of various colours terminating on the splayed walls which gently curve to the focal point, the proscenium opening. With a plain surround, this was flanked on either side by three narrow plaster columns contrasting in white, whilst concealed lighting effects added lustre to the draperies. Behind the proscenium the stage was the full width of the theatre and 25ft. in depth, below which the area at ground level was utilised for dressing and store rooms.

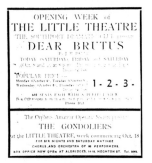

The decorations were described as pleasing and restful, green being the predominant colour, with seats in green upon a flooring of two-tone green Wilton carpet. The entrance hall and winding staircase were fitted with green marble patterned linoleum, relieved by cream shaded walls with subdued concealed lighting. The area was furnished with rust and fawn Axminster carpets, natural oak chairs covered in rust hide and oak tables with pastel green tops. All the windows were furnished with pelmets and curtains of green leaf damask giving a restful atmosphere.

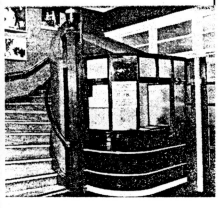

The modern Little Theatre was a far cry from the St Andrews Church Hall where 24 years previously the club was founded, and with the exception of the war years has been the home of the S.D.C. for over 45 years. The outbreak of World War II in 1939 resulted in the almost immediate dispersal of the active membership to the war effort, and the theatre was then hired by the Sheffield Repertory Co., whose own theatre was closed. The S.D.C. moved back in 1946 giving their first public amateur production for over seven years on 7th November with Dodie Smith's *Dear Octopus* which ran for nine evenings to almost capacity audiences.

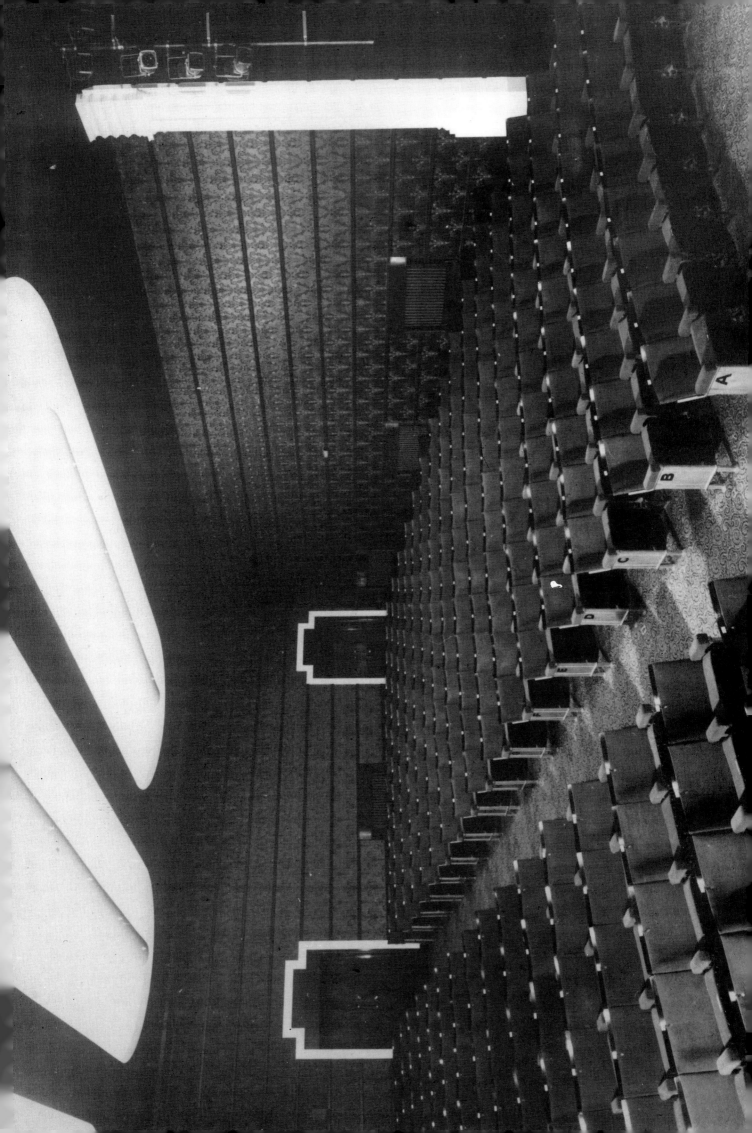

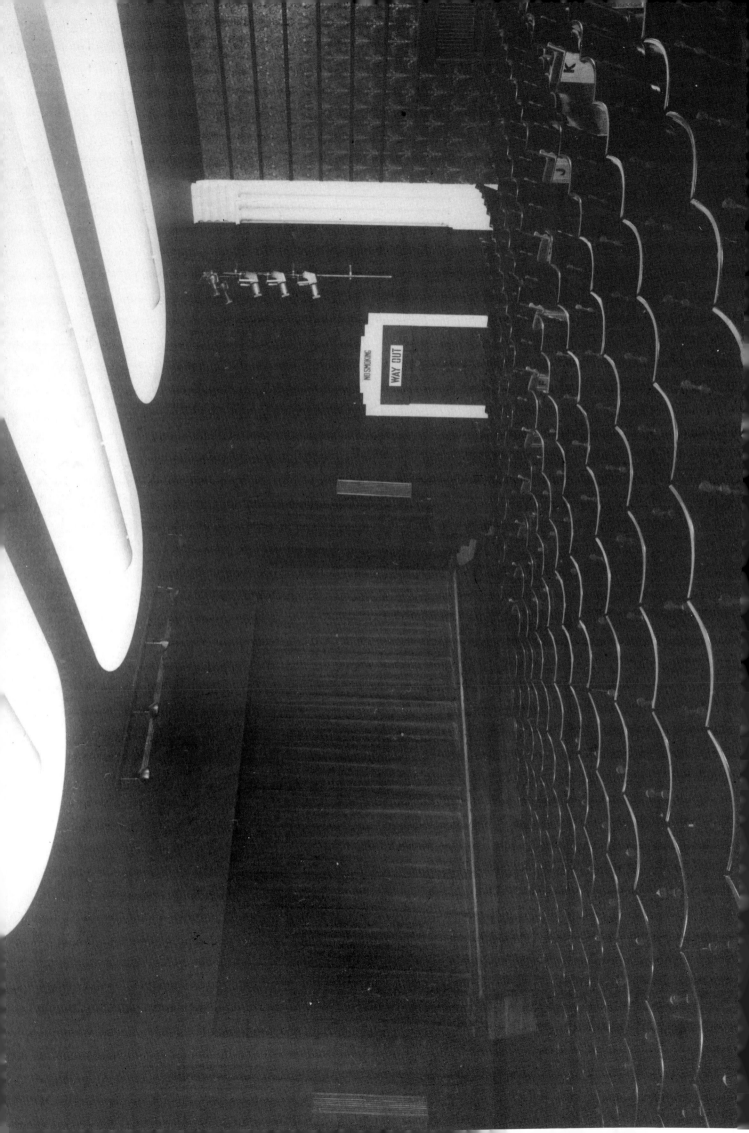

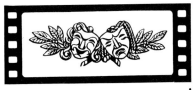

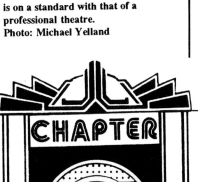

The auditorium of the Little Theatre is on a standard with that of a professional theatre.
Photo: Michael Yelland

During the fifties the success of the club continued to increase, and an audience record was created in 1957 when *The Teahouse of the August Moon* ran to a capacity audience during its eight-night run, and this has since been equalled on other occasions.

In 1966 the club expanded its premises by the acquisition of a house in Scarisbrick Street only 30 yards from the rear of the theatre, which the members transformed into an excellent rehearsal room known as the Little Annexe. A more recent addition has been a licensed bar, reached by a stairway leading down from the foyer, and with the exception of the period of closure due to fire damage at the stage end in December 1987, the Little Theatre has continued to date as a popular rendezvous for the resort's theatregoers.

GRAND CINEMA, Lord Street, Southport

For Southport's cinemagoers, 1938 was a notable year since it saw the opening of two luxury super-cinemas. The first of these, although by only a few weeks was the Grand, at the northern end of Lord Street, where since 1923, the site had been occupied by what was known as Dicky Woodhead's garage, in front of which was a car showroom. The cinema was built as a wedding present for Mrs C. Wood by her husband Mr R.P. Woodhead, who for personal reasons changed his name to Wood, and they were co-directors of the company which they formed, Grand Cinemas (Southport) Ltd.

The architect, George E. Tonge, FRIBA, had by that time, planned many of Southport's entertainment houses, but in designing the facade to the cinema it was an architectural problem to combine the new portion of the front with the old car showrooms. This however was achieved with such success that it was difficult to detect the new part of the frontage from the original of 1923. As in the case of the previously erected cinemas of Lord Street, the appearance was enhanced by the laying out of ornamental gardens by the corporation in front of the building.

The wide frontage was constructed entirely of white faience tiles, which also formed pilasters extending up to the top of the first-floor windows, and below the canopy, divided the main entrance into three ways, each with two pairs of doors surmounted by a window below the canopy, which was set quite high. This had a single row lettering display on the face and a soffit brightly illuminated by neon tubes, which were also used to give prominence to the pilasters after dark, and to the upper part of the frontage, featuring in the centre the large neon sign of the cinema name - GRAND. The three pairs of doors in the main entrance gave access to a spacious foyer, of which decorative fluted columns were a feature. The central column had a bowl terminate with hidden lighting, also concealed lighting in a rectangular recess in the ceiling and eight domes which provided restful illumination. A circular motif gave distinction to the ornamentation of the foyer in colours of light green and cream, which was introduced into the floor covering of multi-coloured rubber.

Flanked on either side by a pay-box, an imposing staircase 12ft wide, in the centre, divided to left and right covered by rich, warm-toned carpet and with specially designed handrails in chromium leading up to the rear of the auditorium and the large cafe with accommodation for 100, decorated in colours of green and silver with fluted columns terminating in elaborate decorative plaster grilles.

There were also entrances to the auditorium through two large side openings in the foyer which gave access to tastefully designed and decorated corridors with large cloakrooms and six illuminated display cabinets. The corridors curved round to the entrance doors at either side of the auditorium where a crossover gangway separated the front stall seats on a raked floor from those up to the rear on a stepped flooring. The covering throughout was by Wilton carpet with a pink pattern on fawn. An indication of the large area is provided by the fact that there were 1,650 large type luxurious seats, widely spaced between the rows, arranged in three sections across, with four gangways illuminated by lights fitted to end seats. The proprietors stated that every seat was of the same type and quality, only the position in the theatre governing the price of admission. An unusual feature of the auditorium was the construction along the side walls of balconettes, on which were fitted seats in pairs, extending to just beyond the front stalls entrances. But it was on entering the theatre at the rear by one of the three entrances that the first impression of the beautiful architecture was obtained. The eye was immediately attracted to the artistically patterned fibrous plaster grilles extending along the curved

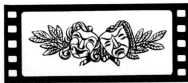

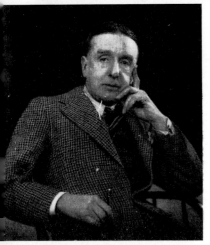

walls flanking the proscenium, and to the massive gold-finished dome in the centre of the ceiling within a circular motif adorned by sixteen stars. This was illuminated by lighting concealed within the dome, the facing of which received light from a central bowl fitting. The grilles served the dual purpose of outlet for the organ music, also ventilation, and were lit with changing colours by neon tubes, as also the large fluted panel above the proscenium, set within a recessed area above the front stalls. The stage curtain was of orange satin, relieved at the lower part by a colourful floral border, which, when illuminated by the footlights exhibited a rainbow range of colours. This opened to reveal the festooned screen curtains of silver satin.

In front of the stage was the organ well, with, in the centre, a lift upon which the Compton console with changing colours, rose to stage level for the organ interludes, and equipped with the Melotone Sound Unit it was stated to provide tonal effects ranging from those of a mighty cathedral organ to a dance band.

Decoration in the art deco style of the '30's was described as bright but not gaudy. At the front, an extension of the gold-edged proscenium formed an attractive setting for the exits, and the toilets, incorporating the electric signs - WAY OUT/LADIES, WAY OUT/ GENTLEMEN. Beyond which, up to the same level, the walls were covered with panelled woodwork in walnut. All other surfaces were treated in broad horizontal bands of colour, sprayed with plastic paint in a gold and green speckled effect, banded with gold and blue.

The projection room, described as one of the finest and most spacious in the north was equipped with Kalee Eleven projectors with sound by the new Western-Electric "Mirrophonic" system, stated to be the greatest advance in sound reproduction since the company introduced "talkies" in 1929.

In addition to the use of cloakrooms free of charge, other amenities were a car park adjoining the theatre, deaf-aid sets for those with defective hearing, and an urgent message service.

An impressive 28 page brochure marking the opening included addresses by the directors, the general and booking manager, Leonard H. Chant and the architect George E. Tonge, all extolling the virtues of the new luxury cinema, which it was stated would bear comparison with any cinema in the North.

The Grand cinema was officially opened at 2.30pm on Monday, 14 th November 1938 by the Mayor of Southport, Councillor W. Geldard, J.P., accompanied by the Mayoress, and on the stage also were the directors, Mr. R.P. Wood, J.P., Mrs C. Wood and the general manager, Mr. Leonard Chant. The opening ceremony was attended by members of the Town Council, magistrates and many other prominent townspeople. The

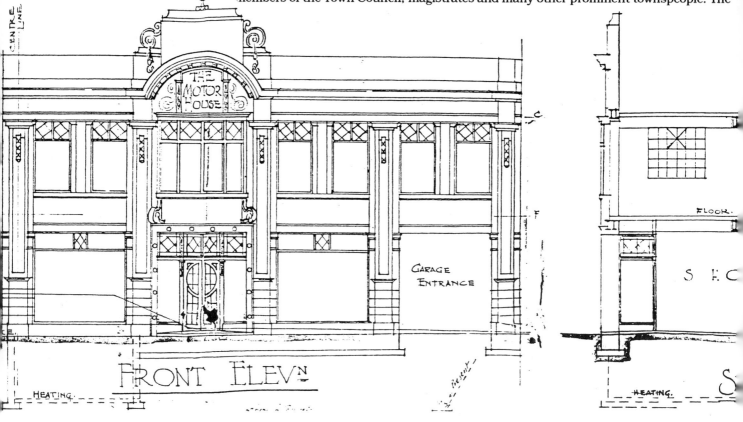

FRONT ELEVⁿ

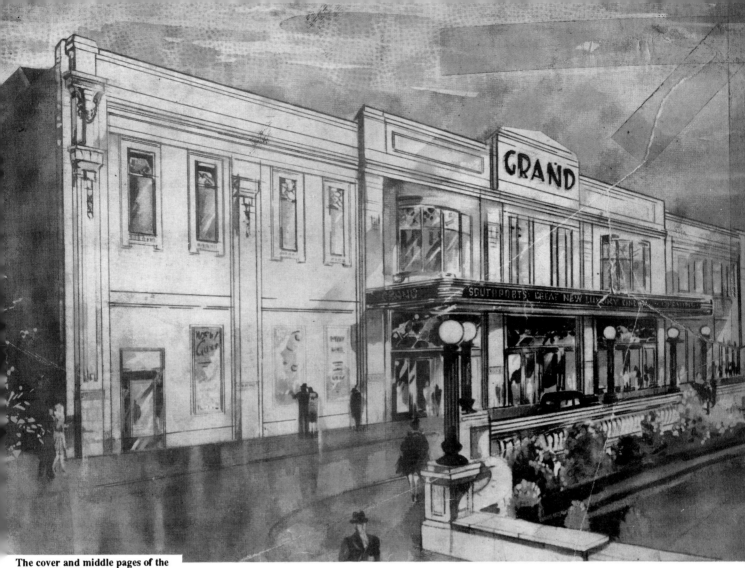

The cover and middle pages of the opening programme.
Collection: L. Houghton

PROGRAMME

1 NATIONAL ANTHEM

2 OPENING CEREMONY
BY HIS WORSHIP THE MAYOR OF SOUTHPORT
COUNCILLOR WILFRID GELDARD

3 GRAND CINEMA NEWS
PRESENTING WORLD EVENTS AS CAMERAS AND
COMMENTATORS CATCH THEM

4 SIT TIGHT—HERE'S THE SCREEN'S
GREATEST NOVELTY
THE NEW AUDIOSCOPICKS

5 INTRODUCING
HERBERT A. DOWSON
AT THE
GRAND COMPTON ORGAN

ARTHUR ★
TRACY
(THE STREET SINGER)
IN

FOLLOW YOUR STAR
WITH
BELLE CHRYSTALL
AND HORACE HODGES

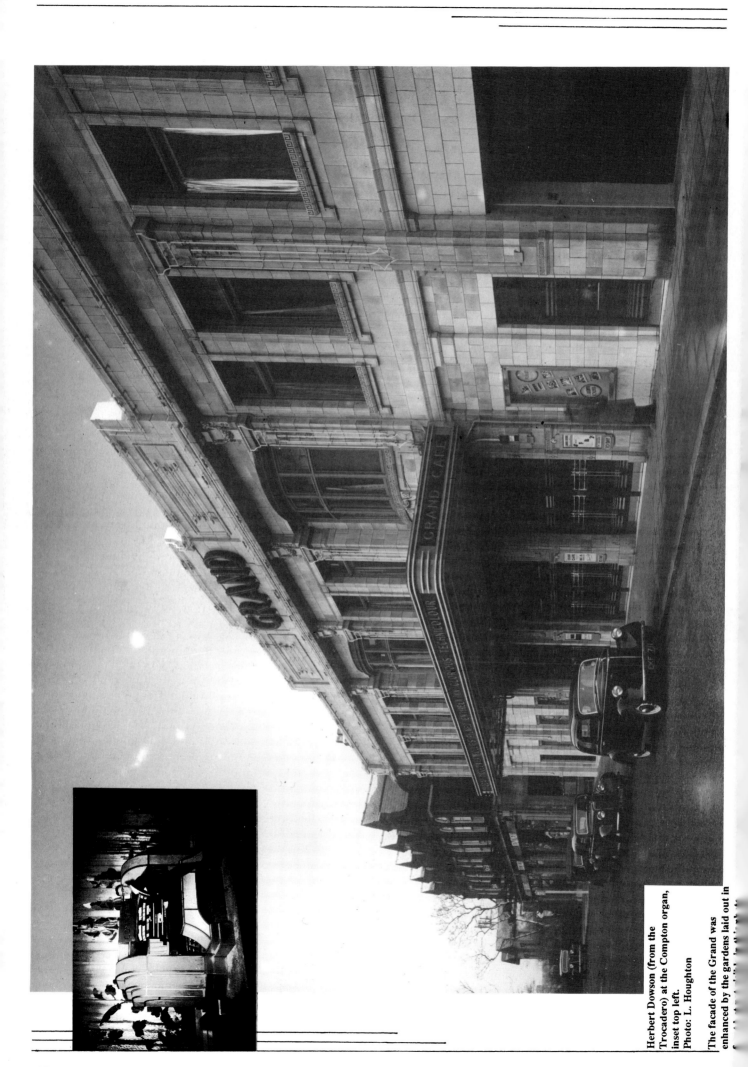

Herbert Dowson (from the
Trocadero) at the Compton organ,
inset top left.
Photo: L. Houghton

The facade of the Grand was
enhanced by the gardens laid out in

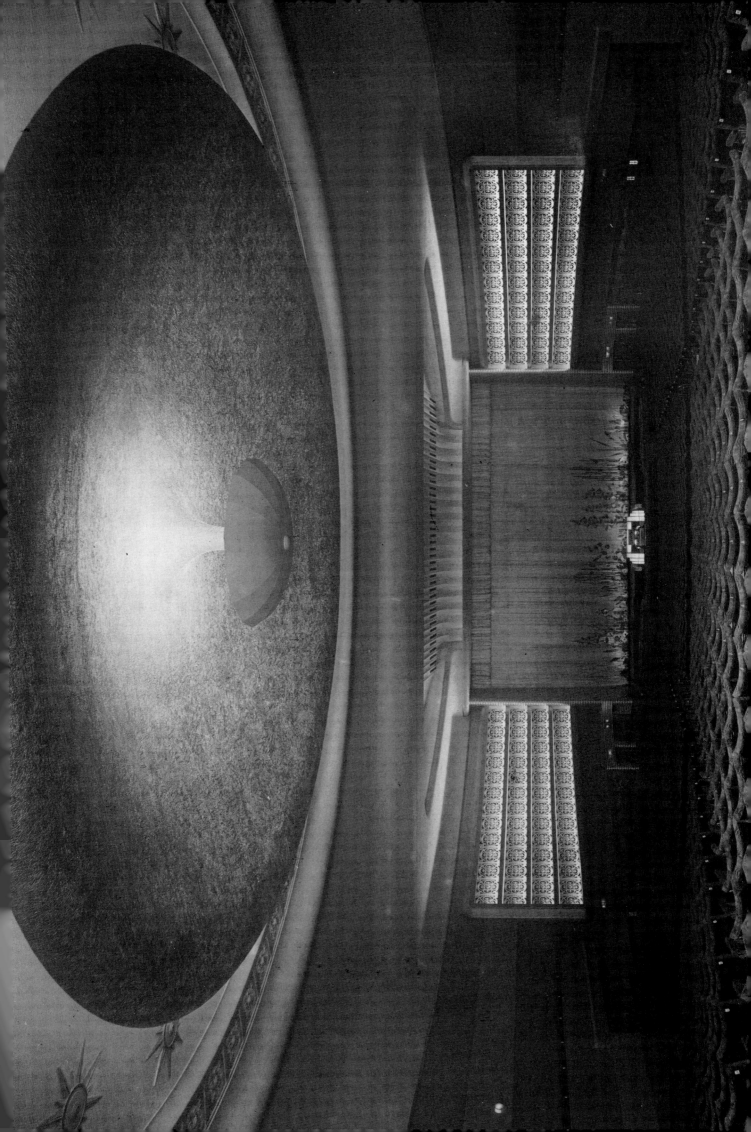

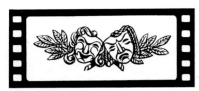

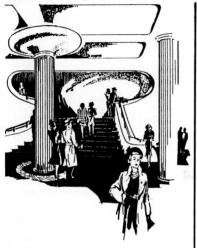

STAIRWAY in MAIN HALL

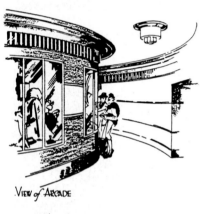

VIEW of ARCADE

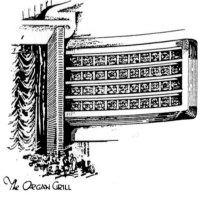

The ORGAN GRILL

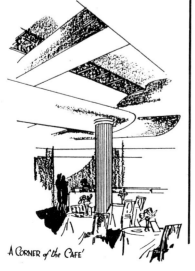

A CORNER of the CAFE

event was recorded on film and included the Mayor's speech, "shots' of the audience and scenes outside the cinema where crowds of people indicated the great public interest in the new venture. It was announced that the film would be shown at all performances during the following week.

Following the opening ceremony the film programme commenced with a newsreel, styled as *Grand Cinema News*, then a novelty film *The New Audioscopicks* after which the illuminated Compton organ console rose for the interlude by Herbert A. Dowson, who four years previously had been Southport's first broadcasting organist. The feature film was *Follow Your Star* featuring Arthur Tracy (The Street Singer) and Belle Chrystall, who had promised to attend the opening but was prevented by certain circumstances from doing so, and an apology for her absence was made from the stage by Mr. Chant.

The company announced a policy of three performances daily at 2.30pm, 6.30pm and 8.50pm also one performance on Sundays at 8.15pm, with all seats bookable free of charge, except the 6d pit stalls, for the prices of 1/- in the stalls, 1/6d and 2/- in the rear part, styled as Grand Stalls and Royal Stalls respectively.

Although then Southport's finest luxury cinema with standards of comfort and facilities unsurpassed by any cinema in the North, the Grand, under independent ownership faced a great amount of competition in the town, but principally from the Gaumont British theatre, the Palladium, and circuit opposition further increased after only three weeks, when another super cinema, the Regal was opened by Associated British Cinemas Ltd. With opposition from the two major circuits, the number of first-run films available to the Grand was somewhat restricted. From the early forties, first-run films were mainly those of Odeon release consisting of Paramount Pictures and the Odeon split of Twentieth Century Fox and Universal, also British films released by General Film Distributors.

In 1954, CinemaScope provided, even though temporarily, a boost for the fortunes of the Grand, when the proprietors were among the many independents to join the Fox or 4th circuit, securing first-run in the town of Twentieth Century Fox CinemaScope pictures, by installing the full CinemaScope equipment including magnetic stereophonic sound. This was completed in October 1954, but surprisingly, since the Grand was by far the superior cinema, the same arrangement had been made six months earlier at the Trocadero, which had been taken over by Grand Cinemas Ltd. during the 1940s. The Grand opened with CinemaScope on 10th October 1954 showing *Three Coins in the Fountain* starring Dorothy Maguire and Clifton Webb, and gradually took over from the Trocadero, the Fox CinemaScope releases until the late fifties by which time the dispute between Twentieth Century Fox and the Rank Organisation had ended with the result that first-run of this producer's films appeared at the Gaumont.

The shortage of first-run films in the sixties began the decline of the Grand, and the cafe, leased by the well-known northern caterers, Reeces, closed c1965. The cinema continued with mainly second-run films and re-runs, and in 1963 the Compton organ was removed to Cheetham Hill Methodist Church, Manchester, but during the past few years has been located at the Chorley Town Hall. In 1966 a Compton organ illuminated console of a similar type from the Regal, Douglas, Isle of Man was installed at the Grand, and for a short time Charles Smart was the resident organist, but following the change to bingo, it was played by William Hopper, the former organist at the Gaumont, until the year before his death in 1978.

The organ console remains *in situ* but covered over and unused for a considerable time.

Decreasing attendances in the large capacity auditorium eventually resulted in closure on 2nd July 1966 when the final programme was a very long double feature comprising re-runs of *Thunderball* featuring Sean Connery as James Bond, also Peter Cushing as Sherlock Holmes in *The Hound of the Baskervilles*.

The Grand was then acquired by Mr. George James, the chairman of the James Casino group and his son Mr. John James, who two years previously had opened the sucessful Kingsway Casino club on the promenade. Since the mid-eighties, the Grand bingo club and Casino have continued under the control of Granada Theatres Ltd.

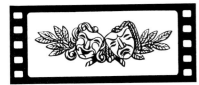

A night view of the Grand, showing the effect of floodlighting and neon. The auditorium shows the luxurious auditorium which was considered the finest in the North, not just in Southport.
Photos: L Houghton

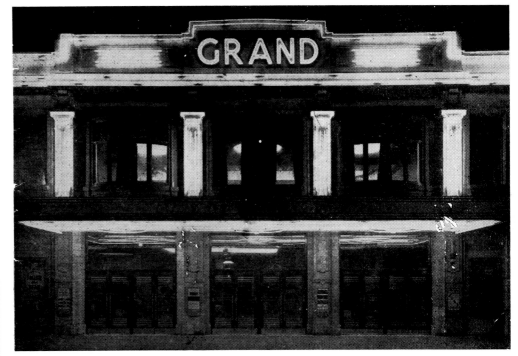

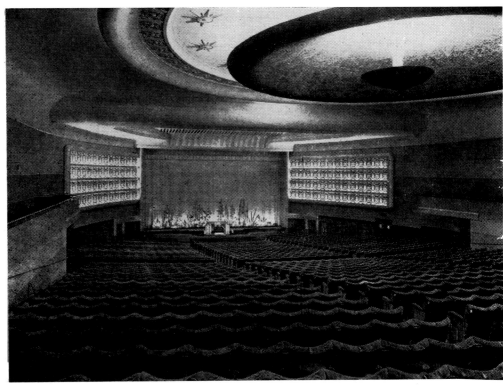

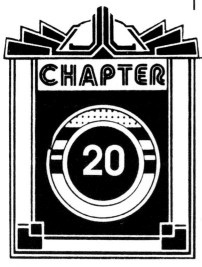

CHAPTER

20

REGAL/ABC CINEMA, Lord Street.

Only three weeks had passed since the opening of the Grand Cinema when in December 1938, the Regal, another luxury super-cinema was a further admirable addition to the town's places of entertainment. Erected at the junction of Lord Street and Wellington Street this was the latest enterprise of Associated British Cinemas Ltd., whose architect W.R. Glenn, FRIAS. supervised the construction by Messrs Frank Haslam Ltd., the builders of several other northern cinemas.

The length of the building being parallel to Lord Street provided a long main frontage of cream glazed faience tiles relieved by brickwork and tall glazed architectural features whilst the side elevation was similarly treated. The right-hand side of the frontage at which was sited the main entrance was given prominence by the exclusive use of tiles as also

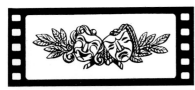

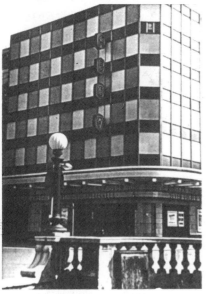

In the 1960s the facade was covered in two-tone blue panels and the name changed to ABC.
Photo: Mike Taylor

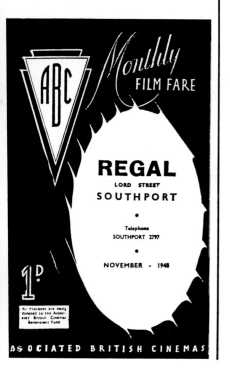

along an adjoining part of the side elevation. Curving at the corner, the full length canopy extended along this with a single row lettering display on the facia, and further advertising for the current attraction was provided immediately below the canopy by a two-row wall-mounted lettering display. Attractive stills frames were fitted by the main entrance and along the main frontage. Illumination of the lower part of the frontage was by neon tubes on the soffit of the canopy, whilst above, the tall glazed areas were internally illuminated and near to the corner at the highest point of the frontages, the cinema name signs were outlined by neon tubes below which the company advertised ownership by the familiar ABC triangles.

Three pairs of glass panelled doors in the main entrance gave access to the spacious foyer with central 'island' pay-box overlooked by the circle lounge, the front of which formed a bridge with metal balustrade linking the stairways at either side of the foyer. Extending forward at a great height, the lounge ceiling surmounted a deep plaster frieze whilst in the centre, attractively patterned mouldings formed a suitable setting for the suspended chandelier light fittings.

Access to the stalls was via a waiting room at the rear of the foyer with advance booking office on the left, beyond which two pairs of doors led onto the rear crossover gangway. Four gangways across the auditorium divided the seating into three blocks providing accommodation for 964 patrons. Extending considerably over the stalls, the circle had a seating capacity of 668 in which the front seats were separated from those of the rear by a crossover gangway reached from the circle lounge at the left and right via doors at the foot of a short flight of stairs. To facilitate the rapid clearing of this part of the auditorium, in addition to two exits at the rear, a short extension at either side led to two exits adjacent to the flanking proscenium walls.

The wide proscenium was adorned by a gold festooned curtain relieved by a scattering of flowers in various colours, and flanked on either side by a broad fluted column beyond which the splayed walls featured elaborate gold painted grilles above the front stalls exits. Above the proscenium a large grille was incorporated on the curve of the ceiling extending to a trough from which it was illuminated by concealed lighting. This was also fitted in the troughs above the circle extending to the rear, and at either side additional lighting was provided by glass shaded light fittings. At the rear of the circle the large projection suite extended over the rear crossover gangway, and was supported by broad square columns. As at the majority of ABC cinemas, Ross projectors and arcs with sound by the R.C.A. Photophone system were installed, the proprietors stating that expense had been a minor consideration in ensuring the perfect enjoyment of picture and sound by the patrons.

Despite the indication by the grilles flanking the proscenium that a pipe organ was to be installed, this did not prove to be the case, and the only interludes at the Regal were given on a Hammond electronic organ by Reginald Porter-Brown in the late fifties, a temporary attraction which at that time also toured the ABC cinemas in the Liverpool area.

Representing the latest method in cinema construction and bringing added architectural beauty and charm to the south end of Lord Street, where it had enabled the Corporation to complete yet another link in the scheme of boulevards, the Regal was officially opened by the Mayor, Councillor W. Geldard on the evening of 5th December 1938 in the presence of a "full house" which included members of the Town Council, magistrates and many representatives of the town's business and social interests. For an hour prior to the opening ceremony, fashionably dressed crowds were constantly arriving in the flower bedecked entrance hall. There was also a charming blaze of floral magnificence in front of the stage, from which the opening ceremony was performed. The Mayor was accompanied by the Mayoress, and Mr. A.S. Moss, general manager of Associated British Cinemas Ltd., who as Chairman, following speeches from the stage, took the opportunity of introducing to the audience the Regal's manager, Mr. Lionel Durban Long, a leading showman of considerable experience in the position, who during the previous three years had been in charge of the company's Capitol Cinema, Bolton.

Following the singing of the National Anthem, the Mayor and Mayoress and party were conducted to seats in the circle for the programme of films in which the main feature was *Vivacious Lady* starring Ginger Rogers and James Stewart, also supporting programme including *Pathe Super Sound Gazette*. After the close of the performance, the principal guests were entertained at the Prince of Wales Hotel by the directors of ABC where a supper was followed by dancing.

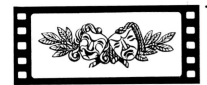

Performances at the Regal originally consisted of a matinee, Monday to Saturday at 2.30pm, separate evening shows at 6.30 and 8.45pm and one performance on Sunday at 8.15pm. Stalls seats were at 6d and 1/- whilst admission to the circle was at 1/6d and 2/-, all bookable in advance except for the front stalls.

As at many leading cinemas, early closing by 10pm during the war years resulted in a change to continuous performances throughout the day, a policy which continued up to the time of decreasing admissions in 1975.

With principal competition from Gaumont British, (succeeded by Rank) also three local independent companies, the Regal played first-run of all ABC circuit release films, some of which during the summer seasons were pre-general releases. Since prospective patrons had little or no information about these films, this was not always an advantage, which went to the independent taking second run.

The early fifties was a time of decreasing cinema admissions and in 1953 the Regal presented the first of the new techniques designed to bring back the missing patrons, this was known as 3-D, three dimensional pictures. But to obtain the effect, patrons had to wear the special spectacles handed to them at the pay-box when purchasing their tickets. The first of these films at the Regal was *House of Wax* featuring Vincent Price, followed by *Phantom of the Rue Morgue*, *The Charge at Feather River* and finally *Kiss Me Kate* in March 1954. By this time the novelty of 3-D had faded, and was followed by the wide screen system, CinemaScope, for which the Regal's proscenium opening was ideally suited. It was only the second cinema in the town to be so equipped, although minus the added attraction of magnetic stereophonic sound as at the Trocadero. The Regal opened with its first CinemaScope film *The Command* starring Guy Madison on 26th August 1954.

The Regal continued as a single-screen cinema until closure, internal improvements being of re-decoration and re-seating which reduced the capacity to 1,488. During the sixties the exterior was considerably changed due to the deterioration of the faience tiles by salt air erosion. The principal area above the entrance was covered by a glazed composition in squares of light and dark blue relieved by narrow horizontal sections in black. Upon this was fitted vertically the four internally-illuminated units of the ABC lozenge-type display sign, the cinema like many others of the circuit having been re-named the ABC. In the centre of the facade was fitted a large internally-illuminated changeable-lettering display advertising the current programme.

In 1969 the old Ross projectors and RCA sound equipment were removed for the installation of Philips DP 75, 70/35mm projectors and Dolby stereo sound, with which the first public performance took place on 12th June 1969 with the 70mm re-issue of *Gone With The Wind*.

But despite the improvement in projection and sound in addition to the more comfortable seating, attendances continued to decline, and in 1975 it became necessary to reduce running costs by part-time opening with continuous evening shows and matinees normally on Monday, Thursday and Saturday only.

Apparently the proprietors, then Thorn-EMI, did not consider the option of conversion to two or more screens justifiable in this situation, for they applied to the Sefton MBC for a change of use to a bingo and social club. Planning permission was granted, but a bingo licence was subsequently refused due apparently to the objection of Ladbrokes, who then controlled the "Lucky Seven" bingo club in the former Garrick Theatre, directly opposite on Lord Street.

The ABC then continued for a further nine years as a single screen cinema with declining attendances, normally in the circle only.

In 1984 a firm of property developers made application to the council for permission to demolish the building and re-develop the site with a block of flats forming a continuation of the existing flats which had adjoined the cinema for many years. But the future of the building was undecided when Thorn-EMI closed the cinema on 1st September 1984, when at 7.30pm the audience was admitted for the last time for the film *Star Trek III* and a supporting film *Balham, Gateway to the South.*

Thereafter the building was unused for nearly three years, then demolished during the summer of 1987, after which construction soon commenced on the flats which now occupy the site of the former Regal Cinema.

The photos on the following two pages show the imposing frontage and auditorium of the Regal. The heart of any cinema is the projection box, seen here with its complement of Ross projectors and RCA sound equipment.
Photo: Stewart Bale

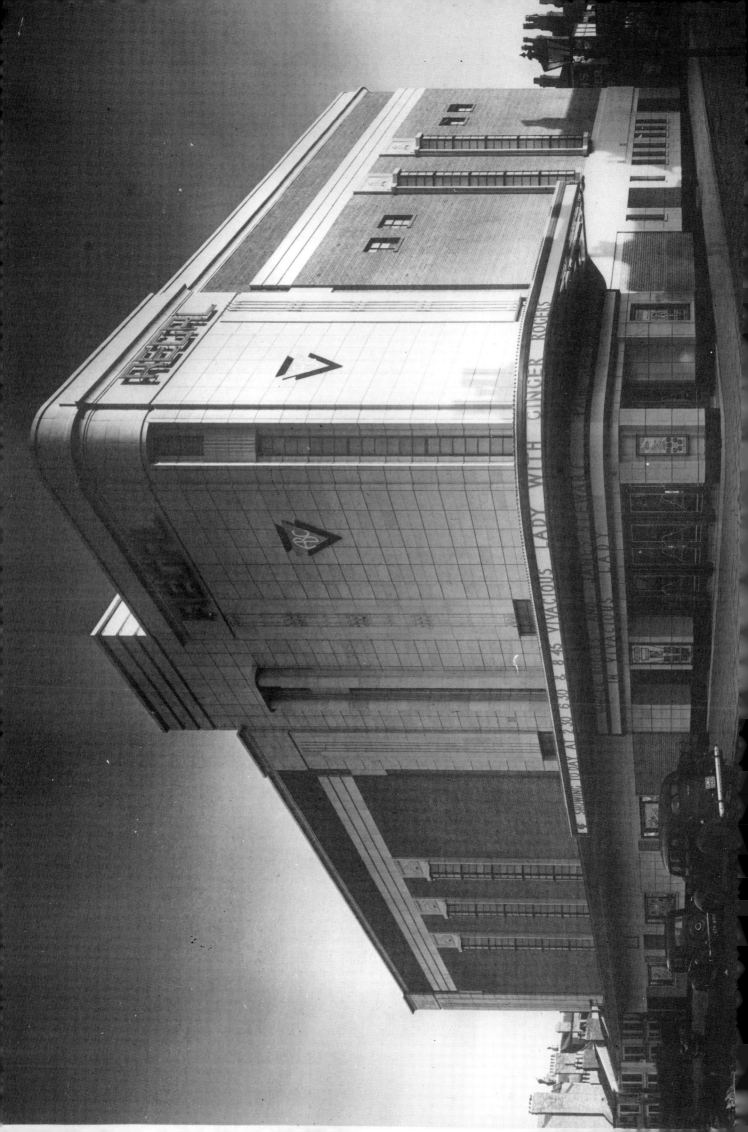

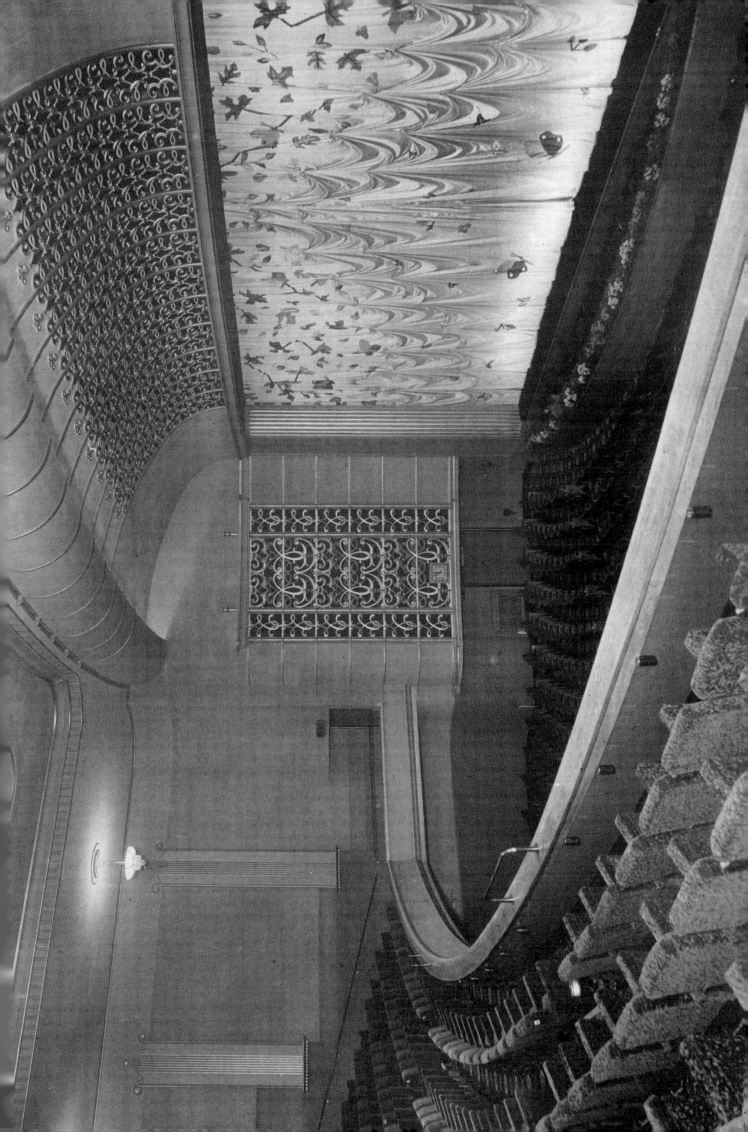

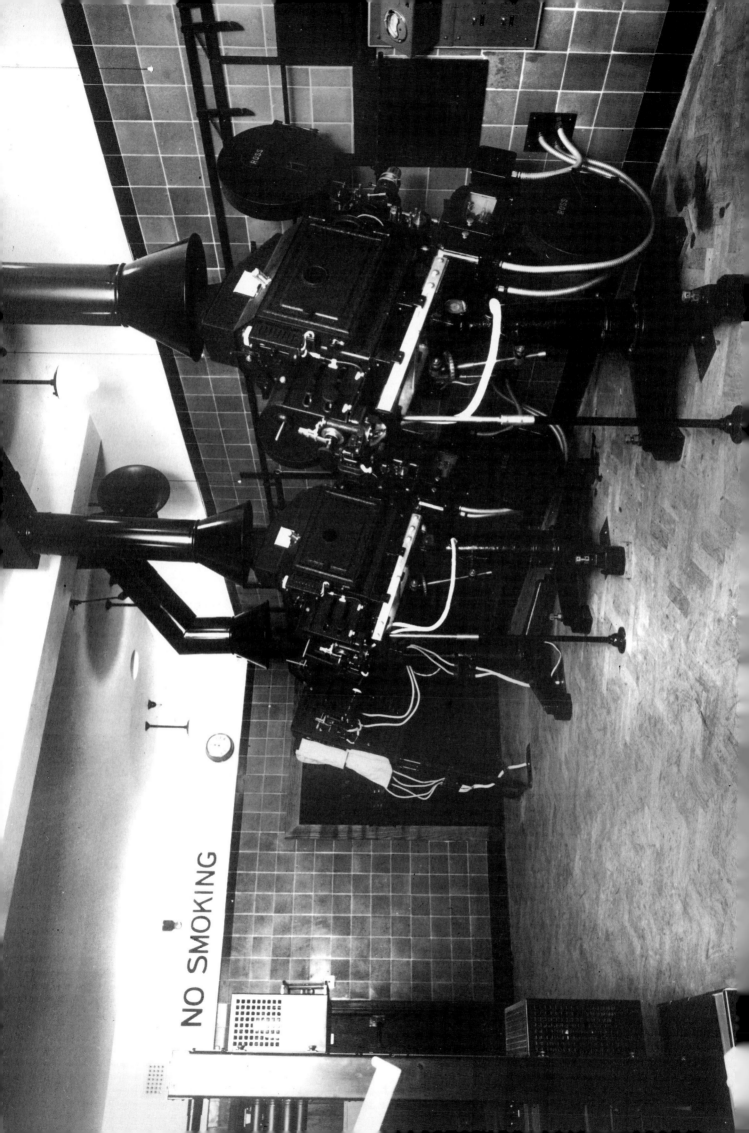

NO SMOKING

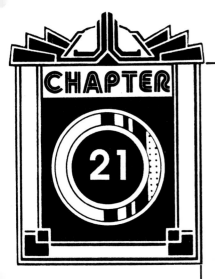

CHAPTER 21

SOUTHPORT THEATRE, Promenade, Southport

Almost a decade after the Garrick Theatre became a bingo and social club, in August 1972, the Southport Corporation announced the plans of architect, Mr. B.R. Andrews of Raikes Construction, Cleckheaton, Yorkshire for a large new theatre which would not only be a fitting venue for international stars, but also serve as a cinema, concert hall or conference centre, in a multi-purpose complex including the Floral Hall.

Construction began in November 1972 and the building was completed in six and a half months at a final cost of £264,000 on the site adjacent to the Floral Hall to which entry was from the new connecting foyer at below ground level. Although eminently suited to the purpose for which it was designed, the new theatre has no special internal or external architectural features, which had been the subject of so much admiration of the older theatres.

Adjacent to the Floral Hall lengthways to the promenade, the construction is of stone relieved by vertical sections of dark brick with splayed areas between the main entrance at the extreme left and the stage block at the opposite end. Surmounted by an advertising display, internally lit by neon tubes, the main entrance with three pairs of doors leads into the carpeted foyer, which extends to the left terminating at the booking offices. Opposite the entrance a broad staircase descends to the spacious foyer with access to the Floral Hall immediately on the left, whilst to the right is situated the licensed bar, sectioned off and furnished with tables and chairs. Beyond this a wide corridor with walls of brick leads to the stairways up to a large area in the centre of the auditorium approximately midway between the stage and the rear, where steps and wooden partitions divide the front portion of the seating from those of the rear on a stepped floor. At the time of opening it was stated that there was seating accomodation for 1,650 people with super comfortable seating and a perfect view of the stage and the cinema screen, but for events requiring a smaller auditorium, the front portion could be separated by a curtain. The plain style of decoration was relieved by a pleated fabric covering the splayed sections of the side walls whilst the seats of the front and rear in deep cerise and pinkish lilac respectively, were described as elegantly contrasting with each other and the remainder of the decor.

The stage was considered versatile, since it was possible to increase the depth by a large apron extension instead of the conventional orchestra pit. No footlights were therefore provided, and the stage is illuminated from overhead battens and spotlights in the projection room at the rear of the auditorium. The plans provided for the auditorium to be equally suited for use as a cinema, for the proscenium, approximately 50ft. in width accommodated the 43ft. wide screen, a size which at the time of opening was desirable for the best presentation of wide screen films in Todd AO and CinemaScope, with a picture 'throw' of 150ft. from the projection room.

Offering an unrivalled choice of entertainment backed up by bar and restaurant facilities the new theatre apparently had every chance of success, The Southport Corporation announced the Gala Opening on 23rd May 1973 when the opening ceremony was performed by Alderman Harold Barber, Chairman of Publicity and Attractions. The star artiste of the performances at 6.30pm and 9.15pm was Marlene Dietrich with full London Orchestra under the direction of William Blezard and arrangements by Burt Bacharach. Seats were bookable at a great range of prices from £1.10s to £3.

The following month was allocated to the leading film attractions "On the Giant Screen" commencing on 4th June with *Man of La Mancha* featuring Sophia Loren and Peter O'Toole, and followed by other wide screen films such as *Ryan's Daughter* and *Kelly's Heroes*.

During the remainder of the seventies the entertainment continued with star variety including a special show during the summer season and a pantomime at Christmas whilst many other dates were allocated to films.

In 1980 came the surprise announcement that the theatre had made a loss of a quarter of a million pounds, a situation which gradually appeared to lead to the ceasing of the summer season star variety shows which by the mid-eighties were replaced by one-night big name shows, This entertainment, together with a pantomine at Christmas and quite frequent use as a cinema continues to date.

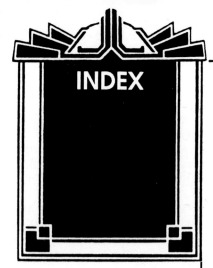

INDEX

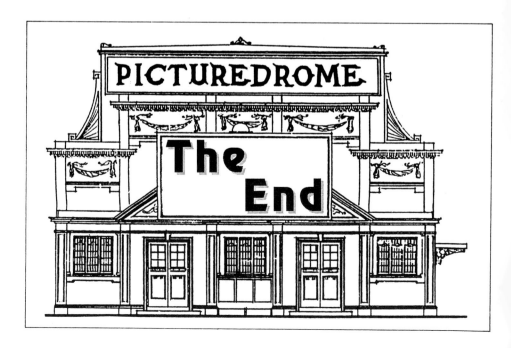

This book is number *223*
of a limited edition of 450.

Signed

Amber Valley Print Centre